OXFORD MEDICAL PUBLICATIONS

Imaging in paediatrics:
a casebook

Imaging in paediatrics: a casebook

Kieran McHugh

Consultant Paediatric Radiologist, Oxford Radcliffe Hospital NHS Trust, Oxford

Oxford   New York   Tokyo
OXFORD UNIVERSITY PRESS
1997

Oxford University Press, Great Clarendon Street, Oxford OX2 6DP

Oxford New York
Athens Auckland Bangkok Bogota Bombay Buenos Aires
Calcutta Cape Town Dar es Salaam Delhi Florence Hong Kong
Istanbul Karachi Kuala Lumpur Madras Madrid Melbourne
Mexico City Nairobi Paris Singapore Taipei Tokyo Toronto

and associated companies in
Berlin Ibadan

Oxford is a trade mark of Oxford University Press

Published in the United States
by Oxford University Press Inc., New York

A catalogue record for this book is available from the British Library

Library of Congress Cataloging in Publication Data
McHugh, Kieran.
Imaging in paediatrics : a casebook / Kieran McHugh.
(Oxford medical publications)
Includes bibliographical references and index.
1. Pediatric diagnostic imaging.   2. Pediatric diagnostic imaging–
–Examinations, questions, etc.   I. Title.   II. Series.
[DNLM: 1. Diagnostic Imaging–in infancy & childhood.   WN 240
M478i 1997]
RJ51.D5M33 1997   618.92′00754–dc20   96–34709
ISBN 0 19 262776 7 (Hbk)

Typeset by EXPO Holdings, Malaysia
Printed in Great Britain by The Bath Press

To Alison.

Preface

This book has been written primarily for paediatricians in training prior to the MRCPaediatrics examination. It should also be found useful by medical students during their paediatrics rotation. Radiology trainees may benefit from reviewing the 100 sets of images and from the clinical information contained within each case. The book may also enable paediatricians in general to 'freshen up' their radiological skills.

The 100 images encompass the whole range of paediatric radiology as it is currently practised with particular emphasis on plain radiology. Few cases of trauma to the paediatric skeleton have been included as trauma plays a small role in medical paediatric examinations. Ultrasound is of fundamental importance in the imaging of children but it is essentially a dynamic process that does not lend itself to the blind interpretation of single images and so not many ultrasound images have been used in this book. The role and usefulness of ultrasound has been repeatedly stressed throughout the text, however.

A question and answer format has been used as this is the best and quickest method of preparing for examinations in general. The book has been arbitrarily divided into five sections (neonatology, cardiovascular and respiratory, gastrointestinal and genitourinary, musculoskeletal, and neuroradiology). Candidates for a paediatrics examination should be familiar with the diverse nature of current imaging techniques as applied to children. A basic understanding of and approach to radiological interpretation is included in the text and the layout of the book should allow readers to practise their technique. Some of the clinical and radiological information in the text is brief and simplified as detailed descriptions of the various topics covered is beyond the scope of the book. Readers are referred to the bibliography for more wide-ranging information. One or occasionally two references of relevant radiologic or paediatric interest are also included at the end of each case.

Although many illnesses, particularly in children, can be tragic, the anonymous interpretation of radiographs and other images can be stimulating and enjoyable. Go ahead—enjoy quizzing yourself and improving your knowledge of paediatric radiology. Good luck in the examination. Hopefully, this book will reduce your need of it!

Oxford   K. McH.
January 1997

Acknowledgements

I often suspect that many authors dedicate books to their wives as a matter of form. Not so in this case! My wife, Alison, has had to read and edit every case and others also which have been discarded, and yet modestly refused to be listed as an editor or contributor. I would also like to thank the staff of Oxford Medical Illustration for preparing the illustrations for this book and Allison Greene for typing much of the manuscript.

The following doctors made contributions to the enterprise and their help is gratefully acknowledged. Mike Pike, Peter Sullivan, Ann Thomson, Lucy Grain, Carolyn Adcock, Amanda Ogilvie-Stuart, Peter Hope, Mary Anthony, Kevin Ives, Eugene McNally, Oxford; Susan King, Alder Hey, and David Martin, Buffalo, USA. Finally, I thank Jo Fairhurst, Southampton, for allowing me to use some radiographs from the Wessex Children's Radiology Department Museum.

'and what is the use of a book, without pictures or conversation?'
Alice in Wonderland

Experience is the name every one gives to their mistakes.
Oscar Wilde

Contents

1. Neonatology

Extracorporeal membrane oxygenation
Congenital cystic adenomatoid malformation
Meconium aspiration syndrome
Duodenal atresia
Malrotation with volvulus
Hyaline membrane disease
Lingual thyroid
Pulmonary interstitial emphysema
H-type tracheo-oesophageal fistula
Periventricular leucomalacia
Bronchopulmonary dysplasia
Meconium ileus
Choanal atresia
Congenital diaphragmatic hernia
Meconium plug syndrome
Intraventricular haemorrhage
Hirschprung's disease
Left lung and right upper lobe collapse; endotracheal tube complication
Necrotizing enterocolitis
Oesophageal atresia
Meconium peritonitis

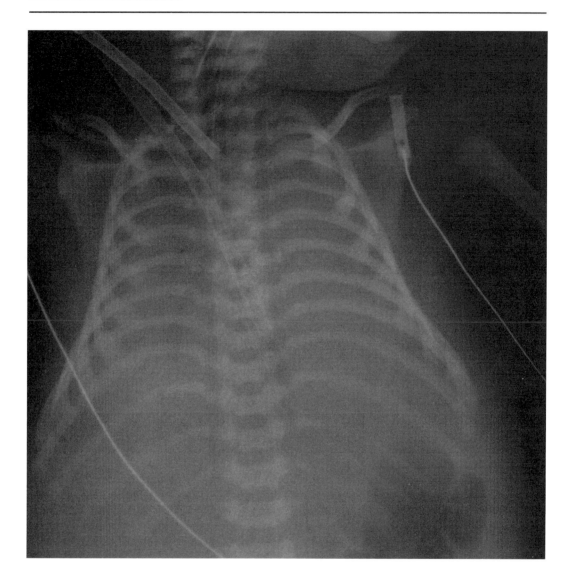

What procedure is this neonate undergoing?

Extracorporeal membrane oxygenation (ECMO)

In addition to an endotracheal (ETT) and nasogastric tube, two larger catheters are evident entering from the right side of the neck. The larger catheters are perfusion cannulas for venoarterial bypass—one is placed in the right atrium via the right internal jugular vein and the other into the common carotid artery so that the tip is at the origin of the innominate artery from the aortic arch. The lungs are opaque, a frequent occurrence while on ECMO. Widespread oedema is present in this patient with thickening of the subcutaneous tissues of the chest wall.

ECMO is used to support infants with severe respiratory and/or cardiac failure unresponsive to conventional therapy. Venoarterial or venovenous (with a double lumen cannula in the right heart) bypass through a semipermeable silicone membrane provides oxygenation and removal of carbon dioxide. ECMO avoids the barotrauma of high inspired oxygen concentration that occurs with ventilation thus allowing the lungs time to heal (10–14 days approximately). All neonates on ECMO have an ETT in place but with mechanical ventilation reduced to minimum levels.

ECMO is commonly used in severe cases of meconium aspiration syndrome, congenital diaphragmatic hernia before and after repair, and neonatal pneumonia. It is generally successful in breaking the cycle of pulmonary hypertension and right to left shunting in these patients. Progressive lung opacification occurs early in almost all neonates on ECMO and is due to a combination of alveolar fluid accumulation, atelectasis, and pleural effusion.

Gross, G. W., Cullen, J., Kornhauser, M. S., and Wolfson, P. J. (1992). Thoracic complications of extracorporeal membrane oxygenation: findings on chest radiographs and sonograms. *Am. J. Roentgenol.*, **158**, 353–8.

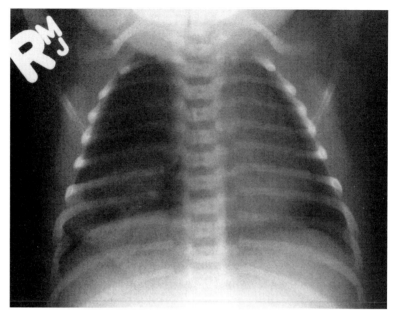

(a)

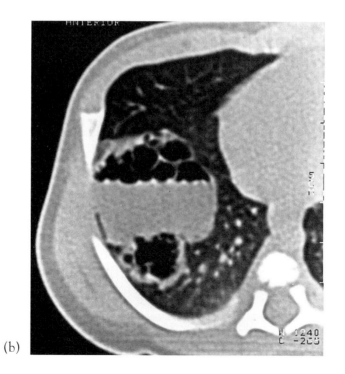

(b)

What lesion is present in the right lower lobe on the chest radiograph and CT in this neonate with respiratory distress?

Congenital cystic adenomatoid malformation (CCAM)

A large opacity is present in the right lower zone within which there is an ill-defined rounded translucent area. The CT confirms a mass lesion with multiple air-filled cysts typical of a CCAM.

CCAM results from the anomalous development of terminal respiratory structures which leads ultimately to the formation of communicating cysts of varying size. It is generally classified into three subtypes. Type I contains large cysts often greater than 2 cm in diameter; in type II malformations smaller cysts are found. Type III lesions have solid adenomatoid tissue with no macroscopic cysts and frequently have other congenital, particularly renal, anomalies in association. Type III lesions have a poor prognosis with maternal hydramnios and foetal hydrops frequently present antenatally.

In type I malformations the cysts are fluid-filled during the first few days of life and the mass appears solid on plain radiographs. Normal bronchial communications are lacking but air later enters the cysts via anomalous channels. Presentation can be within a few hours or months of birth with respiratory distress or in early childhood with recurrent pneumonias. Type I CCAM has the most favourable prognosis, usually being cured by surgical excision.

The differential diagnosis of air-filled cysts or mass lesions on a neonatal chest radiograph includes congenital diaphragmatic hernia, CCAM, sequestration, or pneumatoceles from a resolving staphylococcal pneumonia.

Deacon, C. S., Smart, P. J., and Rimmer, S. (1990). The antenatal diagnosis of congenital cystic adenomatoid malformation of the lung. *Br. J. Radiol.*, **63**, 968–70.

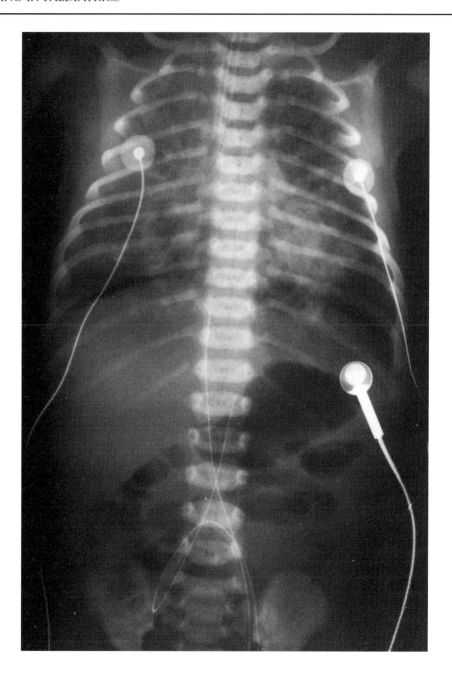

1. What are the two most likely causes of the pulmonary abnormalities in this newborn?

2. Two catheters are seen coursing through the abdomen—which needs repositioning?

1. (a) Meconium aspiration syndrome (MAS)
*   (b) Neonatal pneumonia*

2. Umbilical arterial catheter

There is widespread coarse shadowing in both lungs with scattered atelectasis, emphysematous areas at the bases and more confluent consolidation in the right upper lobe. The umbilical arterial catheter, which is identifiable by the characteristic loop through the iliac artery in the pelvis, has its tip at the L1 level i.e. approximately at the origins of the renal arteries. To prevent renal thromboembolic complications in particular, the catheter tip should be repositioned either below L3 or in the lower thoracic region. The other catheter in the abdomen is an umbilical venous catheter.

MAS occurs as a result of intrauterine aspiration of meconium. It is seen most frequently after intrapartum asphyxia, predominantly in postmature infants. The effect of meconium aspiration on the lungs is essentially a combination of mechanical obstruction of the major airways and a chemical pneumonitis more peripherally.

The radiographic features of MAS depend largely on the severity of aspiration. Patchy infiltrates with areas of overinflation and atelectasis are typically seen in severe cases, occasionally with a pleural effusion. Air leak phenomena such as a pneumothorax or pneumomediastinum are common complications. However, MAS can be indistinguishable from neonatal pneumonia due to Group B streptococcal infections as the findings in both conditions can be extremely variable.

Wood, B. P. (1993). The newborn chest. *Radiol. Clin. North Am.*, **31**, 667–76.

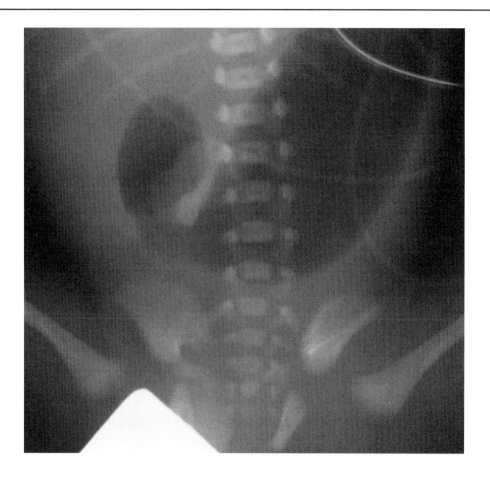

What is the diagnosis on the abdominal radiograph of this neonate?

Duodenal atresia

There is gaseous distension of the stomach and proximal duodenum causing the classical 'double-bubble' sign of duodenal atresia. The rest of the abdomen is gasless.

Duodenal atresia occurs in one in 6000 births and up to one third of patients have Down's syndrome (trisomy 21). An antenatal history of polyhydramnios is frequently associated. On antenatal ultrasound a dilated stomach and duodenum suggests the diagnosis which can be confirmed postnatally. Complete duodenal obstruction secondary to atresia becomes symptomatic immediately after birth usually with bilious vomiting as the majority of atresias occur immediately distal to the ampulla of Vater.

The diagnosis is confirmed by an abdominal radiograph often after a small amount of air has been injected via a nasogastric tube. Contrast studies are rarely necessary and may be hazardous because over-filling of the stomach with complete duodenal obstruction poses a high risk of gastro-oesophageal reflux and associated pulmonary aspiration.

Lee, F. A., Mahour, G. A., and Gwinn, J. L. (1978). Roentgenographic aspects of intrinsic duodenal obstruction. *Ann. Radiol.*, **21**, 133–42.

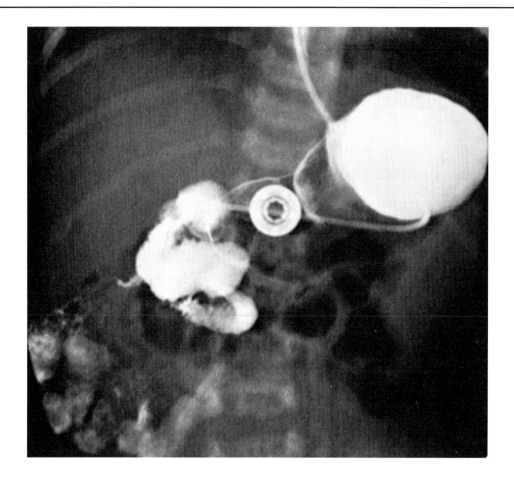

What is the diagnosis on this contrast meal examination in a three-day-old boy with bilious vomiting?

Malrotation with volvulus

The proximal duodenum is dilated and partially obstructed. The duodeno–jejunal flexure (DJ) is abnormally positioned in the midline and the proximal small bowel loops are right-sided.

Malrotation encompasses a wide variety of anomalies of intestinal rotation and fixation. The DJ flexure which indicates the position of the ligament of Trietz should normally be located to the left of the midline at the level of the gastric antrum. The normal, broad-based small bowel mesentery extends from the left upper quadrant to the right iliac fossa. When the ligament of Trietz and caecum are poorly fixed a short mesentery predisposes to midgut volvulus. The gut can twist around the superior mesenteric artery (SMA) leading to bowel ischaemia and ultimately necrosis. Malrotation with volvulus usually presents in the neonatal period with bilious vomiting but can be intermittent and delayed presentation in later childhood is well recognized.

Bilious vomiting, with or without small bowel loop dilatation on abdominal radiographs, should always alert the clinician to the possibility of malrotation in a child. A contrast or barium meal should be performed urgently to assess the nature and level of obstruction. Identification of the position of the DJ flexure is critical in the diagnosis of malrotation. When a volvulus is present the proximal small bowel can have a corkscrew appearance on the contrast study as its twists around the SMA. A contrast enema, by defining the position of the caecum, is an alternative method of diagnosing malrotation but an upper gastrointestinal study is generally more reliable. Ultrasound, by demonstrating anomalous positioning of the SMA and superior mesenteric vein, can occasionally be suggestive of malrotation, but the diagnosis ultimately is dependent on the findings on a contrast study.

Long, F. R., Kramer, S. S., Markowitz, R. I., *et al.* (1996). Intestinal malrotation in children: tutorial on radiographic diagnosis in difficult cases. *Radiology*, **198**, 775–80.

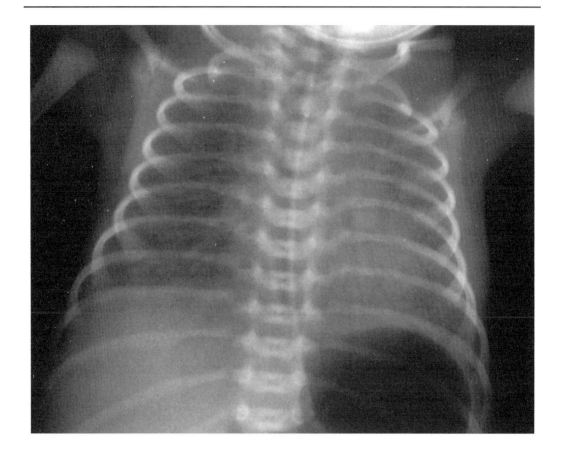

What is the diagnosis in this premature infant?

Hyaline membrane disease

Symmetrical ground-glass shadowing or lung granularity bilaterally typical of hyaline membrane disease is evident. Faint air bronchograms with loss of clarity of the cardiac and diaphragmatic contours are visible.

Hyaline membrane disease (HMD) is due to a deficiency of pulmonary surfactant which results in alveolar collapse. Although essentially a disease of prematurity, other risk factors for HMD include perinatal asphyxia, caesarean section, and maternal diabetes. The chest radiography will usually be abnormal by six hours with the maximum radiographic changes seen around 24 hours of age.

Fine reticular shadowing or granularity is initially evident progressing to lung white-out with air bronchograms, lung hypoaeration, and loss of clarity of the diaphragmatic and cardiac contours. The radiologic hallmark of hyaline membrane disease is symmetrical granularity in both lungs but after treatment with exogenous surfactant or ventilation asymmetric changes are common. Subsequent acute deterioration, which may be indistinguishable from HMD, can be caused by pulmonary haemorrhage or left to right shunting across a patent ductus arteriosus, although in the latter condition cardiac enlargement may be evident. Neonatal infection which often causes asymmetric lung shadowing, can also have an identical radiographic appearance to HMD. For this reasion antibiotics are routinely administered in many neonatal units for at least the first 48 hours of life until the results of the first blood cultures are negative.

Poulain, F. R. and Clement, J. A. (1995). Pulmonary surfactant therapy. *West J. Med.*, **162**, 43–50.

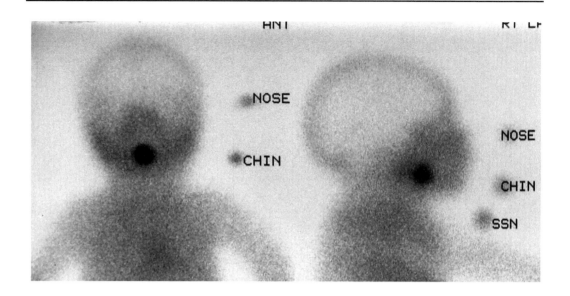

What abnormality is evident on the radionuclide thyroid study in this infant with congenital hypothyroidism?

Lingual thyroid

There is intense focal uptake of Tc99m-pertechnetate in the posterior aspect of the mouth, typical of a lingual thyroid. No functioning thyroid tissue is visible in the neck (SSN = suprasternal notch).

Congenital hypothyroidism can result from defective thyroid gland embryogenesis, defective synthesis of or responsiveness to thyroid hormone, hypothalamic–pituitary abnormalities, and intrauterine exposure to goitrogenic drugs. Hypoplasia or dysplasia of the gland may be associated with thyroid ectopia. The majority of cases of a lingual thyroid are picked up on newborn screening programs although thyroid ectopia does not always result in hypothyroidism. Occasionally ectopic thyroid tissue first manifests in later childhood or near puberty with an enlarging mass at the base of the tongue.

Tc99m-pertechnetate is used in thyroid scintigraphy as pertechnetate ions are trapped by the thyroid in a similar manner to iodine through an active transport mechanism. Sonography can easily identify a normal thyroid gland in the neck but provides no information regarding thyroid function and is less sensitive than scintigraphy in identifying thyroid ectopia.

Wells, R. G., Sty, J. R., and Duck, S. C. (1986). Technetium 99m-pertechnetate thyroid scintigraphy: congenital hypothyroid screening. *Pediatr. Radiol.*, **16**, 368–73.

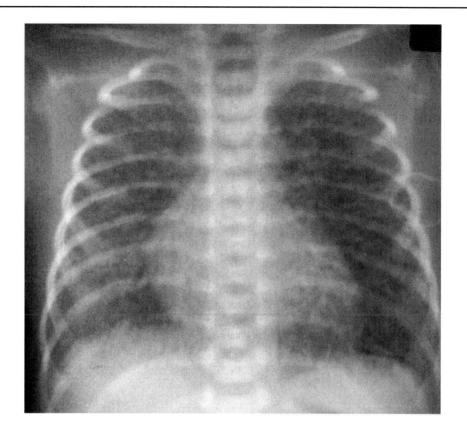

This five-day-old neonate has been ventilated for hyaline membrane disease. What complication has occurred?

Pulmonary interstitial emphysema (PIE)

The lungs are hyperinflated with multiple small cystic radiolucencies present bilaterally due to interstitial emphysema.

PIE is predominantly seen in preterm babies as a complication of mechanical ventilation for hyaline membrane disease. Alveolar rupture results in air dissecting through the interstitial tissues and lymphatics. The volume of the affected lung is usually increased. The abnormality may be bilateral but is often unilateral with shift of the mediastinum to the contralateral side. A pneumothorax is a common complication and should be suspected with sudden unexplained deterioration in the clinical status. An air-leak may also occasionally result in a pneumomediastinum or pneumopericardium.

PIE appearing within 24 hours of birth generally indicates severe underlying lung disease and has a poor prognosis. On plain radiographic appearances alone, larger cysts due to PIE may be difficult to differentiate from the findings in bronchopulmonary dysplasia (BPD), but the former usually arises within the first two weeks of life whereas the changes of BPD generally take three weeks or more to develop.

Cochran, D. P., Pilling, D. W., and Shaw, N. J. (1994). The relationship of pulmonary interstitial emphysema to subsequent type of chronic lung disease. *Br. J. Radiol.*, **67**, 1155–7.

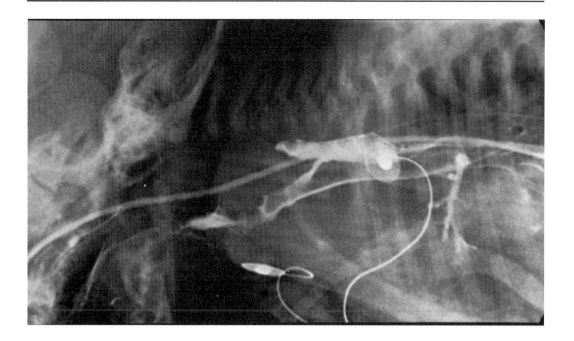

What abnormality is demonstrated on the oesophagogram?

H-type tracheo-oesophageal fistula

The infant has been placed in the prone position with a feeding tube positioned in the distal oesophagus and then withdrawn gradually whilst contrast was injected. An H-type tracheo-oesophageal fistula has opacified with contrast, with spill into the trachea and major bronchi.

H-type fistulae without oesophageal atresia present later than pure oesophageal atresia. Symptoms include choking, coughing attacks or cyanosis during feeding, and recurrent pneumonias.

Plain radiographs are usually normal but may show gaseous abdominal distention and pneumo-oesophagus especially after endotracheal intubation and positive pressure ventilation. The fistula can be difficult to demonstrate on conventional barium or contrast studies. An oesophagogram obtained in the prone position whilst injecting contrast with a feeding tube *in-situ* is the best method of demonstrating an H-type fistula. Oesophagoscopy or bronchoscopy are alternative techniques which are generally reliable in the diagnosis of these fistulae but involve sedation or anaesthesia and a contrast study is the preferred initial diagnostic examination. Commonly there is a solitary fistula at or above the level of the second thoracic vertebra—consequently repair can be achieved via a cervical incision which is considered a safer surgical approach than a thoracotomy.

Kirk, J. M. E. and Dicks-Mireaux, C. (1989). Difficulties in diagnosis of congenital H-type tracheo-oesophageal fistula. *Clin Radiol.*, **40**, 150–3.

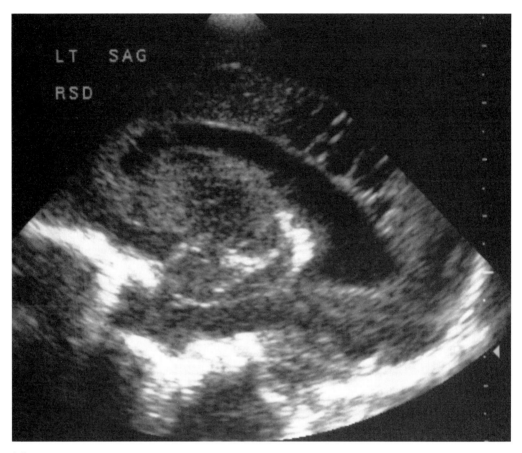

(a)

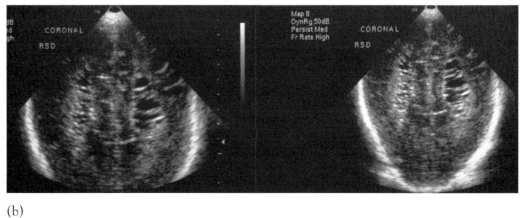

(b)

What abnormality is present on the (a) left parasagittal and (b) two coronal neonatal cerebral ultrasound images?

Cavitating periventricular leucomalacia

Anechoic cavities, typical of periventicular leucomalacia, are seen mainly in the parieto-occipital regions paralleling mildly dilated lateral ventricles.

Periventricular leucomalacia (PVL) results from ischaemic injury to the premature brain. Unlike in term infants, the periventricular regions in the premature are a watershed area between arterial territories and are therefore particularly vulnerable to ischaemic damage. The clinical sequelae of PVL are varied but developmental delay, spastic diplegia, cortical visual impairment, and cerebral palsy may result.

PVL characteristically manifests on cerebral ultrasound as a flare of increased echogenicity adjacent to the lateral ventricles, particularly in the frontal and occipital regions. It is usually a bilateral process. As some periventricular echogenicity is a normal finding, milder degrees of PVL may pass unrecognized. The typical flare of PVL may resolve with time but often progresses to form multiple cavities two to six weeks after the ischaemic episode. Only after cavities develop can PVL be diagnosed unequivocally. Cavitating PVL and multicystic encephalomalacia may appear similar sonographically, but strictly speaking multicystic encephalomalacia can occur in any part of the brain and often results from intraparenchymal haemorrhage.

Babcock, D. S. (1995). Sonography of the brain in infants: role in evaluating neurologic abnormalities. *Am. J. Roentgenol.*, **165**, 417–23.

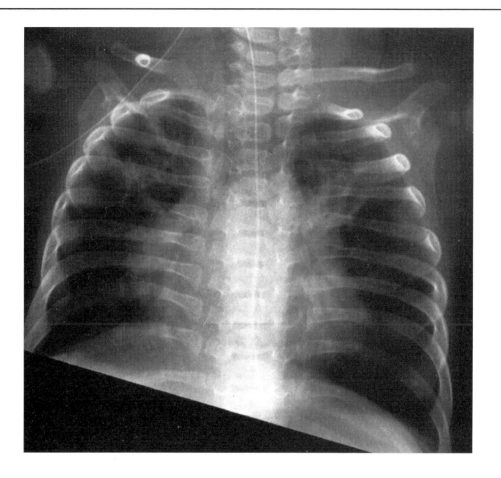

This six-week-old infant was treated for hyaline membrane disease. What condition has ensued?

Bronchopulmonary dysplasia (chronic lung disease of prematurity)

There is coarse streaky shadowing with atelectasis and fibrosis predominantly in the upper lobes with overinflation of the lung bases. The tip of the nasogastric tube is in the distal oesophagus and should be advanced.

Bronchopulmonary dysplasia (BPD) is the term applied to the lung changes seen in infants who most commonly have had prolonged treatment for hyaline membrane disease (HMD). Occasionally BPD follows other neonatal conditions such as meconium aspiration syndrome. Barotrauma from long-term mechanical ventilation with high inspired oxygen tensions ultimately results in areas of emphysematous lung damage, atelectasis, and fibrosis.

Coarse streaky shadowing with patchy overinflation and cystic changes are the classic radiographic findings in BPD (or type 2 chronic lung disease). The usual sequence is that of slow resolution of HMD with gradual change over a few weeks to more coarse, asymmetrical lung shadowing. An increasingly common radiological manifestation now is simply diffuse hazy shadowing in both lungs without focal areas of emphysema (type 1 chronic lung disease). Mucous plugging leading to segmental consolidation is a frequent complication and is difficult to differentiate from true infective consolidation. A number of scoring systems have been devised to evaluate the severity of BPD on chest films but they are of doubtful clinical relevance. However, in general, severe changes on chest radiographs usually indicate a worse prognosis.

Lanning, P., Tammela, O., and Koivisto, M. (1995). Radiological incidence and course of bronchopulmonary dysplasia in 100 consecutive low birth weight infants. *Acta Radiol.*, **36**, 353–7.

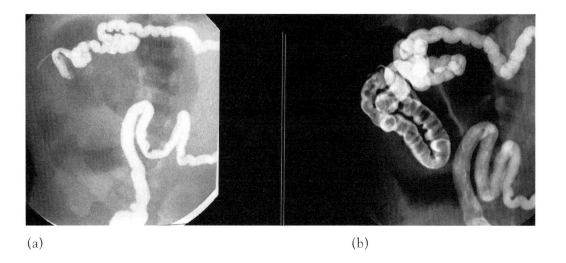

(a)   (b)

These two films are from a contrast enema in a three-day-old neonate with abdominal distension and failure to pass meconium. What is the diagnosis on the enema and the likely underlying disorder?

1. *Meconium ileus*
2. *Cystic fibrosis*

(a) The initial films shows contrast outlining a small colon ('microcolon') with the caecum and appendix visible in the right upper quadrant and no meconium evident in the colon. (b) On the second radiograph taken a few moments later, contrast has passed further retrogradely i.e. into the terminal ileum (which is more distended than the colon had been at the commencement of the study). A large filling defect is present in the terminal ileum due to a cast of meconium. Note gaseous distention of small bowel loops proximally.

Differentiation of large from small bowel obstruction on plain abdominal films in newborns can be extremely difficult. Many suspected neonatal distal intestinal obstructions have a similar clinical presentation. Causes include Hirschsprung's disease, meconium plug syndrome, small bowel atresia, and meconium ileus. All of these four possible diagnoses can usually be confirmed and differentiated by a contrast enema. Moreover, the diagnostic enema for meconium plug syndrome or meconium ileus can be immediately followed by a therapeutic enema. The therapeutic enema is achieved by switching from a standard non-ionic contrast medium to a hyperosmolar medium with the resultant hygroscopic and osmotic effects of the hyperosmolar contrast assisting in the passage of meconium.

A therapeutic enema will relieve the intestinal obstruction in approximately half the cases of meconium ileus; surgery will be required in the remainder. The abnormal thick, viscid meconium causing meconium ileus is virtually always due to cystic fibrosis. However, only 10% of patients with cystic fibrosis present in the neonatal period with intestinal obstruction.

Abramson, S. J., Baker, D. H., Amodio, J. B. *et al.* (1987). Gastrointestinal manifestations of cystic fibrosis. *Semin. Roentgenol.*, **22**, 97–113.

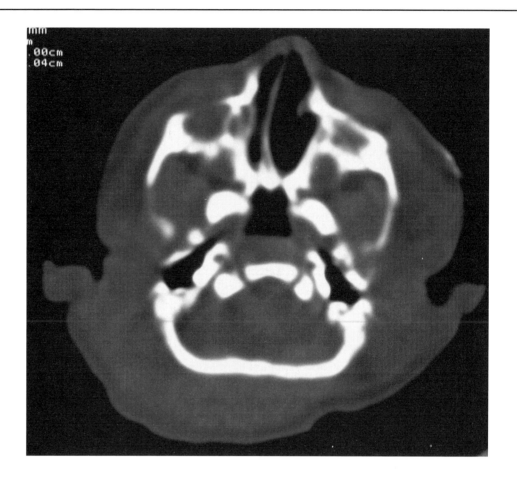

What abnormality is evident on the CT in this newborn who had episodes of dyspnoea during feeding?

Bilateral choanal atresia

Bony choanal atresia is visible in the posterior aspect of both nasal air passages. Note that the lateral walls of the nasal cavity bow medially.

Choanal atresia occurs in 1 in 7000 births, and consists of a bony or membranous septum between the nose and pharynx which may be unilateral or bilateral. Bilateral atresia results in severe dyspnoea during feeds, episodes of apnoea and thick gelatinous mucous in the nasal cavities. The diagnosis is often first suspected when a nasal catheter or nasogastric tube cannot be advanced further than 2–3 cm form the nostril. Unilateral cases are generally not life-threatening and may pass unrecognised. Choanal atresia forms part of the CHARGE association (coloboma, heart disease, atresia of the choanae, retarded growth, genital hypoplasia, ear anomalies).

Fine slice (1–3 mm) CT scanning through the nasal airways has replaced contrast studies as the recommended imaging method for confirming choanal atresia. Prior suctioning is necessary to remove the thick nasal secretions in order to accurately define the membranous type of atresia. The lateral walls of the nasal cavity normally parallel the vomer but typically with all types of choanal atresia the lateral walls are thickened and bowed medially with enlargement also of the vomer.

Prescott CA. Nasal obstruction in infancy. Arch Dis Child 1995; 72: 287–289.

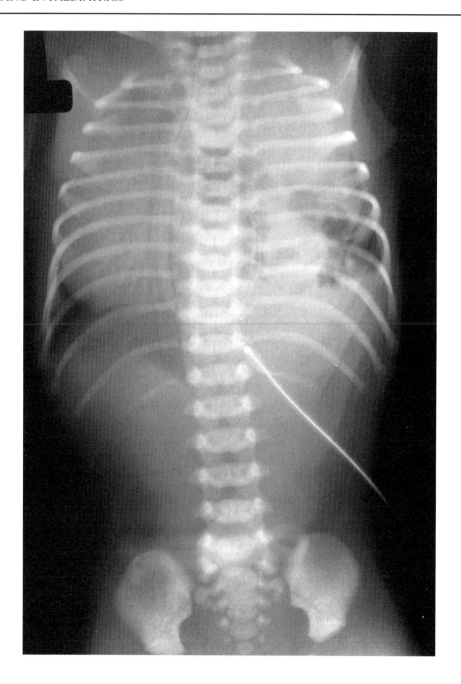

What is the diagnosis?

Congenital diaphragmatic hernia

There is mediastinal shift to the right with abnormal round lucencies at the left base due to bowel gas in the left hemithorax. The nasogastric tube is coiled in the left chest indicating an intra-thoracic stomach. Note absence of bowel gas in the abdomen.

85% of congenital diaphragmatic hernias are left-sided. The incidence is 1 in 3000 births and congenital hernias are generally thought to occur through the foramen of Bochdalek. Although there is increasing antenatal sonographic detection of congenital diaphragmatic hernias, the majority present in the neonatal period with respiratory distress. Occasionally presentation is delayed a few months or years.

Rounded lucencies in the chest due to air in bowel loops which have herniated into the thorax, and mediastinal shift are the characteristic radiographic findings. Absence of bowel gas in the abdomen helps distinguish a congenital diaphragmatic hernia from the two other major causes of rounded lucencies on the chest film in the neonatal period, namely pneumatoceles from a staphylococcal pneumonia and congenital cystic adnomatoid malformation. A pneumothorax contralateral to the diaphragmatic hernia, absence of contralateral aerated lung, and an intrathoracic stomach are features on chest radiography associated with a poor prognosis. The presence of the stomach within the chest may be due to herniation at an earlier stage of gestation resulting in more severe pulmonary hypoplasia. Favourable features on an initial chest X-ray include the presence of aerated lung ipsilateral to the hernia and greater than 50% aeration of the contralateral lung.

Saifuddin, A. and Arthur, R. J. (1993). Congenital diaphragmatic hernia—a review of pre-and postoperative chest radiology. *Clin. Radiol.*, **47**, 104–10.

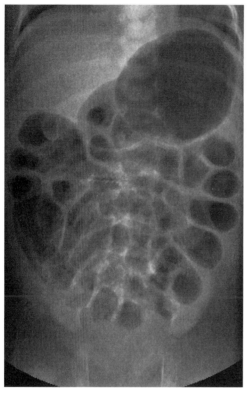

(a)

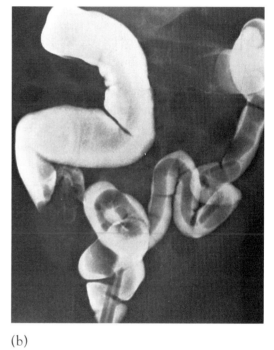

(b)

Plain radiograph and contrast enema in a neonate with abdominal distension and failure to pass meconium. What is the diagnosis?

Meconium plug syndrome (small left hemicolon)

The abdominal films shows gaseous distension of many bowel loops in keeping with a distal intestinal obstruction. On the enema study a cast of meconium is visible as a long filling defect in the descending and sigmoid colon. The colon distal to the splenic flexure is significantly smaller than the transverse and ascending colon which are mildly dilated.

Meconium plug syndrome, small left hemicolon syndrome and functional immaturity of the left colon are similar and probably the same functional disorder of the newborn large bowel. They all result from a non-specific failure of bowel activity presenting in neonates as abdominal distension, bilious vomiting, and/or failure of passage of the first stool. Associated predisposing conditions include prematurity, pre-eclampsia, maternal diabetes, hypothyroidism, and sedation.

A standard contrast enema is curative often with a large cast of meconium being passed immediately after the enema and rapid subsequent improvement. Differentiation from a long segment Hirschsprung's disease with a transition zone at the splenic flexure can be difficult radiologically and all doubtful cases should have suction rectal biopsies. Meconium plug syndrome should also be differentiated from meconium ileus which is an unrelated condition where there is neonatal intestinal obstruction due to inspissated viscid meconium in the terminal ileal region secondary to cystic fibrosis.

Berdon, W. E., Slovis, T. L., Campbell, J. B. *et al.* (1977). Neonatal small left colon syndrome: its relationship to aganglionosis and meconium plug syndrome. *Radiology*, **125**, 457–62.

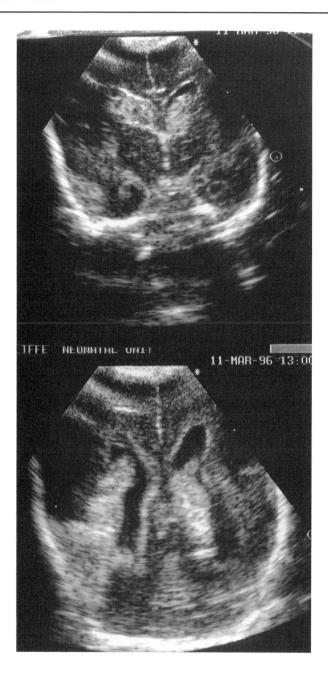

List the abnormalities on the coronal ultrasound images in a premature neonate?

1. *Ventricular dilatation*
2. *Bilateral intraventricular haemorrhage (IVH)*
3. *Intraparenchymal haemorrhage right temporo-parietal area (grade 4)*

The characteristically echogenic choroid is too bulky in this case due to bilateral IVH. The choroid plexus passes inferiorly through the foramina of Monro into the third ventricle and so choroid is not normally seen in the frontal horns of the lateral ventricles. An anechoic area superior to the intraparenchymal haemorrhage on the right is artefactual and not due to porencephaly.

Intraventricular haemorrhage (IVH) and periventricular haemorrhage occur almost exclusively in preterm infants, particularly in those weighing less than 1500 g. The usual site of origin is the germinal matrix in the caudothalamic groove between the caudate nucleus and the thalamus. The germinal matrix is a highly vascular structure which involutes in the third trimester and is not present in term babies.

A frequently used grading system for intracranial haemorrhage is as follows: grade 1, haemorrhage confined to the germinal matrix or subependymal area: grade 2, IVH with normalsized ventricles; grade 3, IVH with ventricular dilatation; grade 4, IVH with adjacent intraparenchymal haemorrhage. Grade 1 haemorrhages are usually of little clinical consequence but the other grades of haemorrhage have a variable but generally increasingly worse prognosis. Severe IVH frequently leads to post-haemorrhagic hydrocephalus. Intraparenchymal haemorrhage initially appears as an area of markedly increased echogenicity adjacent to a lateral ventricle. Large grade 4 lesions typically undergo liquefaction necrosis within a few weeks ultimately leading to the development of an area of encephalomalacia.

Rypens, E., Avni, E. F., Dussaussois, L. *et al.* (1994). Hyperechoic thickened ependyma: sonographic demonstration and significance in neonates. *Pediatr. Radiol.*, **24**, 550–3.

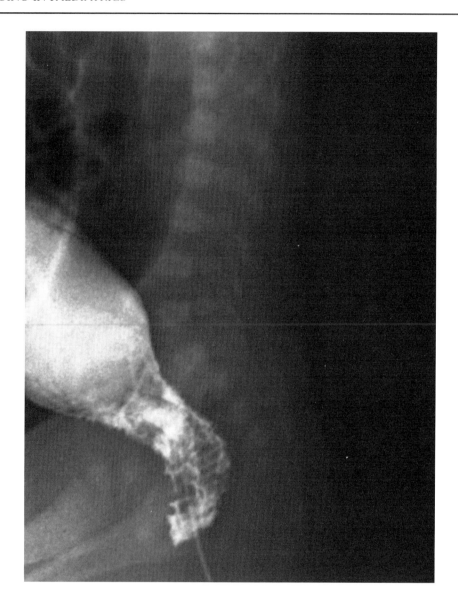

What is the diagnosis seen on the contrast enema of this neonate with intestinal obstruction?

Hirschsprung's disease

There is narrowing of the rectum with a short transition zone between narrowed rectum and dilated sigmoid colon. Abnormal contractions and irregular peristalsis were evident during the study in the narrowed aganglionic rectum, resulting in irregularity to the rectal wall.

In Hirschsprung's disease there is absence of the normal myenteric ganglion cells in the distal bowel with an impairment in peristalsis. Hirschsprung's disease occurs in approximately in 1 in 5000 births. Presentation is commonly in the neonatal period with failure to pass meconium, or constipation, vomiting, and abdominal distension. The area of aganglionosis manifests as hypertonic bowel narrowing and always extends proximally from the anal canal. The transition zone from abnormal to normal ganglionic bowel is located in the rectosigmoid region in approximately 70% of cases.

A contrast enema is useful as an emergency procedure to exclude other causes of bowel obstruction, to identify the length of the aganglionic segment and the likely transition zone which in turn can guide the surgeon to the appropriate site for a temporary defunctioning colostomy. Suction rectal biopsies followed by intraoperative biopsies confirm the diagnosis. Diarrhoea accompanied by rectal bleeding can herald the onset of enterocolitis which is the principal cause of death in Hirschsprung's disease and which may occur even after corrective surgery. Hirschsprung's disease occasionally passes unrecognized in infancy presenting later with chronic constipation in early childhood.

Blane, C. E., Elhalaby, E., and Coran, A. G. (1994). Enterocolitis following endo-rectal pull through in children with Hirschsprung's disease. *Pediatr. Radiol.*, **24**, 164–6.

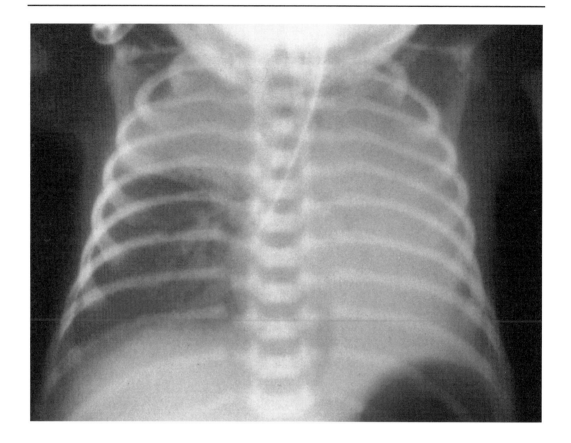

List the abnormalities on the chest film. What is the cause?

1. *Left lung collapse*
2. *Right upper lobe consolidation/collapse*
3. *Endotracheal tube tip in the bronchus intermedius*

The endotracheal tube (ETT) has inadvertently been inserted too far with only the right middle and lower lobes being ventilated. Consequently, consolidation/collapse of the right upper lobe and left lung have occurred. The inferior aspect of the right upper lobe abuts the horizontal fissure and so isolated right upper lobe consolidation has a clearly defined inferior limit on frontal radiographs.

One of the major indications for chest radiography in the paediatric intensive care setting is in the evaluation of the correct positioning and potential complications of the various tubes, catheters, and lines used. Whenever such tubes or catheters are visible on a chest film their placement should always be assessed and noted (see Appendix: Approach to the paediatric chest radiograph).

ET tubes, whether nasally or orally placed, should lie with the tip placed midway between the thoracic inlet and carina. The tube may move with movement of the patient's head. Consequently, an ETT too close to the carina can intermittently slip into the right main bronchus, for example, resulting in inadequate ventilation of the left lung. Similarly, tubes with their tip above C7 have a tendency to become dislodged, particularly in younger children. When an infant's neck is flexed (chin to chest) the tip of the ET tube will move further down the airway and conversely when the neck is extended will rise up to a higher position. Remember: 'chin up, tube up; chin down, tube down'.

Hauser G. J., Pollack, M. M., Sivit, C. J. *et al.* (1989). Routine chest radiographs in paediatric intensive care: a prospective study. *Pediatrics*, **83**, 465–70.

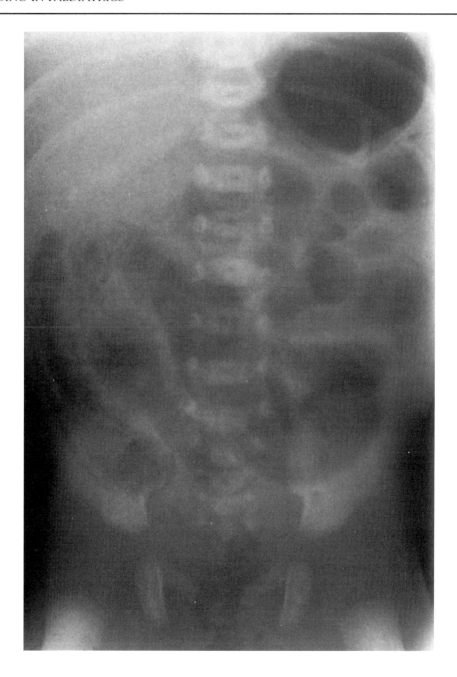

This is a plain abdominal radiograph in a neonate with increased gastric aspirates and bloody diarrhoea. What is the diagnosis? Describe the radiographic findings.

Necrotizing enterocolitis (NEC)

There is distension of a number of bowel loops with scattered intramural gas (pneumatosis intestinalis) typical of NEC. Note the obvious linear pneumatosis of the bowel loop in the right flank. There is no evidence of perforation.

NEC is an acquired condition seen predominantly in premature infants. The onset is generally acute within the first 3 to 4 days of life but can occur at any time between one day to eight weeks. Common presenting features include abdominal distension, bloody diarrhoea, vomiting, increased gastric aspirates, metabolic acidosis, or shock. Early diagnosis and medical management can reduce the need for surgical intervention.

Plain abdominal radiographs are often normal early in the course of NEC such that the diagnosis is made on clinical grounds solely. Dilatation of the bowel and bowel wall thickening are often the earliest radiographic features but are non-specific. A persistently dilated loop of bowel on sequential films is highly suspicious of NEC. With disease progression pneumatosis intestinalis, the hallmark of NEC, becomes evident. Two patterns of pneumatosis may occur: a 'bubbly' pattern due to submucosal air which is difficult to differentiate from stool, and a more easily recognizable linear pattern due to subserosal gas. Transient gas in the portal veins, seen as lucencies in the periphery of the liver, occurs in up to 5% of cases. Perforation is a serious complication that requires surgery and occurs most frequently in the ileo-caecal region. The most common late complication of NEC is stricture formation which is found in approximately 10% of cases, usually in the colon.

Rowe, M. I., Reblock, K. K., Kurkchubasche, A. G., and Healey, P. J. (1994). Necrotising enterocolitis in the extremely low birth weight infant. *J. Pediatr. Surg.*, **29**, 987–90.

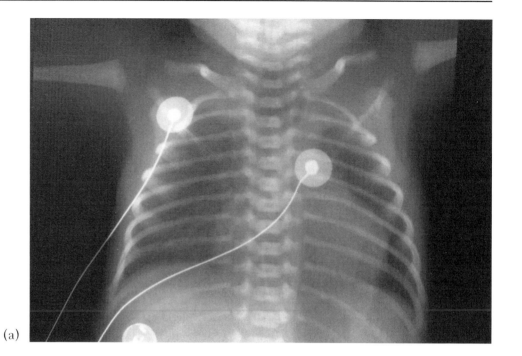

(a)

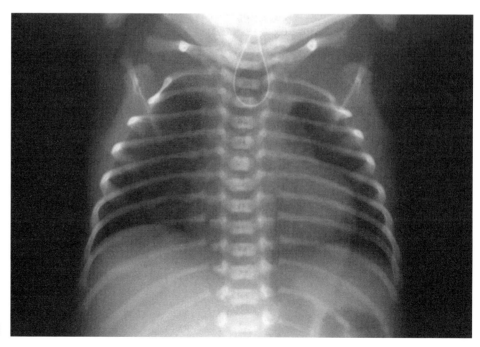

(b)

What is the diagnosis?

Oesophageal atresia

(a) The initial film shows distension of the proximal oesophagus in the superior mediastinum. (b) On the later radiograph a nasogastric tube (NGT) has curled in the proximal oesophageal pouch. Air is present in the gastric fundus. The heart, lungs, and vertebrae are normal. Linear shadows in the left lower zone are due to skin folds.

Oesophageal atresia has an approximate incidence of 1 in 3000 births. There are five major subtypes. The commonest anomaly occurring in about 80% of cases is oesophageal atresia with distal tracheo-oesophageal fistula. Presentation in all cases of oesophageal atresia occurs soon after birth with excessive oral secretions or choking. An antenatal history of polyhydramnios is common. Tracheomalacia due to compression of the trachea by the distended proximal oesophagus is a frequent association. A smaller number of children with oesophageal atresia have the VATER or VACTERL association—often their morbidity and mortality have more to do with the associated renal or cardiac lesions than with their oesophageal atresia.

Failure of passage of a NGT which loops in the blind ending pouch is usually documented by chest radiography. Injection of air can be done via the NGT to distend the pouch and confirm the diagnosis if necessary. Contrast injection should be avoided because of a high risk of pulmonary aspiration. Air in the gastrointestinal tract accumulates via the distal fistula and can lead to marked gaseous abdominal distension particularly in ventilated babies. A right aortic arch is present in 5% of cases and should be sought on frontal radiographs because if detected some surgeons may opt to perform a left thoractomy rather than the usual right sided approach.

In the common oesophageal atresia with distal fistula the gap between the proximal and distal oesophagus is usually short and immediate primary repair is generally possible. A gasless abdomen is the hallmark of oesophageal atresia without a fistula. In patients who do not have a fistula a long gap is frequent, and delayed primary repair allowing growth of the oesophageal segments is common practice.

Spitz, L., Kiely, E. M., Morecroft, J. A., and Drake, D. P. (1994). Oesophageal atresia: at risk groups for the 1990's. *J. Pediatr. Surg.*, **29**, 723–5.

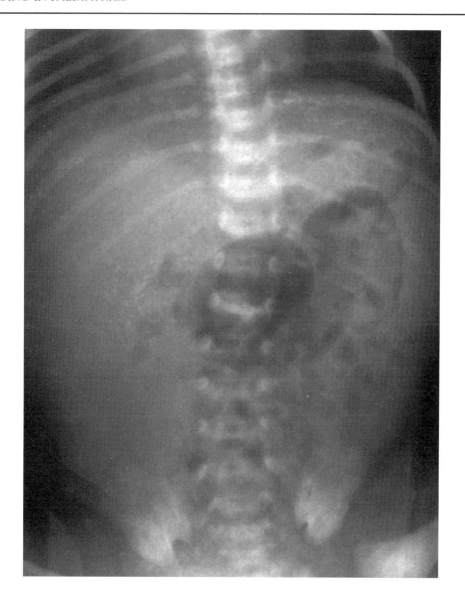

This is a plain abdominal radiograph taken within four hours of birth in a newborn in whom antenatal ultrasound had shown dilated bowel loops. What is the diagnosis?

Meconium peritonitis

There is widespread calcification in the upper abdomen particularly over the liver and in the region of the left hemidiaphragm. One prominent bowel loop is seen centrally over L 1/2 but the bowel gas pattern is otherwise normal.

Sterile meconium leakage into the peritoneal cavity resulting in meconium peritonitis occurs as a result of intrauterine bowel perforation. Calcification within the peritoneum frequently ensues. The usual cause of meconium peritonitis is perforation in association with an intestinal atresia or complicated meconium ileus. Calcification is usually present diffusely within the peritoneal cavity in the former condition but in the setting of meconium ileus secondary to cystic fibrosis the thick, viscid meconium tends not to spread and remains localized, usually in the right lower quadrant.

Absence of dilated bowel loops in the illustration does not entirely rule out an associated intestinal obstruction as the radiograph could have been taken too early for gaseous distension of bowel loops to develop. As a general rule, it takes approximately four hours for gas to reach the caecum after birth in a normal newborn and approximately 24 hours to reach the rectosigmoid region. Interruption of the normal progression of gas through the bowel can be a useful adjunct to the clinical findings in the diagnosis of neonatal obstruction.

Estroff, J. A., Bromley, B., and Benacerraf, B. R. (1992). Fetal meconium peritonitis without sequelae. *Pediatr. Radiol.*, **22**, 277–8.

2. Cardiovascular and respiratory

Bronchiectasis
Empyema
Normal thymus
Epiglottitis
Pneumothorax
Mycetoma
Fallot's tetralogy
Non-Hodgkin's lymphoma
Congenital lobar emphysema
Adult respiratory distress syndrome
Primary tuberculosis
Middle aortic syndrome
Contusion, pneumothorax, subcutaneous emphysema, dislodged tooth
Mediastinal leukaemia
Aspirated foreign body
Cystic fibrosis
Viral pneumonia
Right middle lobe consolidation
Retropharyngeal abscess
Pneumopericardium

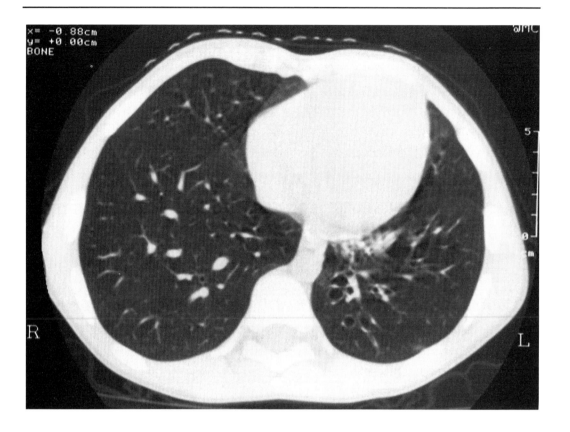

What abnormality is present on this thin slice high resolution CT section through the lower chest in an adolescent with a chronic productive cough?

Bronchiectasis in the left lower lobe

There is dilatation of the bronchi medially in the left lower lobe with associated volume loss. Note the normal right lung with the more anteriorly positioned major fissure (faint linear shadow) separating the right middle lobe anteriorly from the right lower lobe.

Bronchiectasis is a descriptive term for irreversible dilatation of the bronchial tree. While bacterial pulmonary infection accounted for most cases in the past, common causes of bronchiectasis now include cystic fibrosis, immune deficiency, ciliary dysfunction, endobronchial obstruction secondary to aspirated foreign bodies, and childhood viral infections. With the exception of bronchiectasis secondary to an impacted foreign body, it is increasingly being recognized that apparently localized bronchiectatic changes in one lobe are often accompanied by less easily identifiable airway changes elsewhere in the lungs. This, allied to better medical management and physiotherapy, has led to a more conservative approach and fewer indications for surgical resection of bronchiectatic segments.

Plain radiographs are insensitive in the detection of mild bronchiectasis. Dilated bronchi with thickening of peribronchial tissues giving roughly parallel lines, crowding of the bronchi and lobar volume loss are sometimes evident. Thin slice high resolution CT examinations have a high sensitivity in the detection of bronchiectasis and have largely replaced bronchography as the investigation of choice. The normal bronchus is no larger than its accompanying vessel on CT, but in bronchiectasis there is bronchial dilatation often with bronchial wall thickening giving a 'signet ring' appearance. Terms such as cylindrical, saccular or varicose bronchiectasis are frequently used radiological descriptions but are not really helpful in planning management, and suggest a more detailed understanding and classification of bronchiectasis than actually exists (among radiologists at least!).

Kuhn, J. P. (1993). High resolution computed tomography of pediatric pulmonary parenchymal disorders. *Radiol. Clin. North Am.* **31**, 533–51.

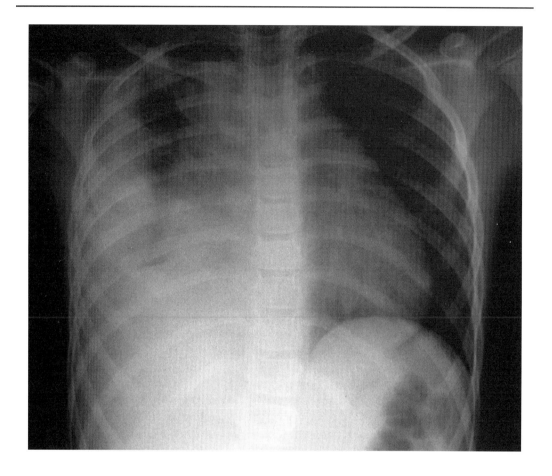

This girl had been treated for a pneumonia for 10 days. What complication has occurred? Describe the radiographic findings.

Empyema

There is a thick band of opacification paralleling the right chest wall with a clearly defined medial margin indicating a large pleural collection. Despite the pleural collection, loss of volume is evident in the right hemithorax with collapse and consolidation in the right middle and lower lobes.

Small effusions are commonly seen in association with bacterial pneumonias and are usually transient. A small pleural effusion is characterized by a thin band of peripheral shadowing paralleling the chest wall often with a curvilinear superior component, the so-called meniscus sign. When an effusion becomes infected an empyema results. Pleural empyemas most often occur secondary to *Staphylococcus aureus*, *Haemophilus influenzae*, and *Streptococcus pneumoniae* infections. It is generally recommended that larger pleural effusions associated with pneumonias are aspirated early, during the exudative phase when the fluid is thin, to prevent empyema formation.

Despite aspiration persistently loculated effusions may occur. Ultrasound examination of the chest can be particularly useful in demonstrating a pleural effusion with associated pleural thickening and areas of loculation, and can act as a guide to indicate appropriate sites for aspiration of loculated fluid. Occasionally empyemas become chronic and organized, and require formal surgical decortication. Prior to surgery CT is often used to assess the degree of thickening of the visceral and parietal pleura, the amount of infected pleural fluid, and to exclude an underlying lung abscess.

Campbell, P. W. (1995). New developments in pediatric pneumonia and empyema. *Curr. Opin. Pediatr.*, **7**, 278–82.

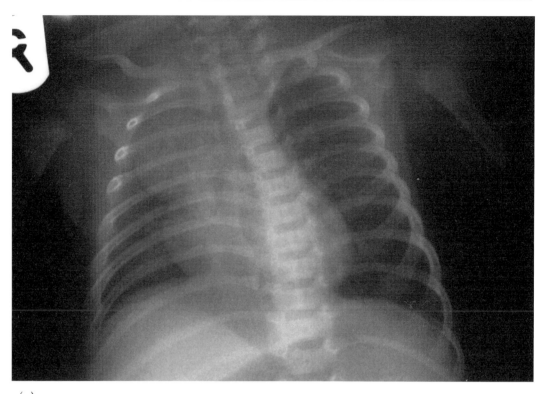

(a)

What is the cause of the right upper zone shadowing on the chest radiograph in this infant?

Normal thymus

The patient is rotated to the right—note prominence of the anterior ribs on the left compared to the right and that the trachea has also rotated to the right. The right upper zone shadowing has a well-defined, rounded inferior margin which could not be due to right upper lobe consolidation. Ultrasound examination of the superior mediastinum showed a normal thymus and no evidence of a thymic cyst or other mass lesion (see Fig. 2.3b).

The thymus in infants and children is a large organ which can extend from the level of the brachiocephalic vessels in the anterior and superior mediastinum to as low as the diaphragm. It is usually visible on frontal chest radiographs up to about four years of age though it can decrease substantially in size during intercurrent illness.

The normal thymus does not compress or displace the trachea and is often sufficiently transradiant on well-penetrated radiographs to allow visualization of normal lung markings through it. The soft thymic tissue often has undulations on its lateral aspect caused by the anterior ribs. The normal thymus tends to have well-defined anterior and inferior borders which are responsible for the so-called 'sail sign'. A prominent thymus can, however, drape itself over and become inseparable from the cardiac shadow and in such cases estimation of the cardiac size can be particularly unreliable.

If there is suspicion that a mediastinal mass may in fact be a normal thymus then ultrasound examination can easily delineate the normal gland. Normal thymic tissue characteristically has homogenous echotexture and does not compress or displace adjacent intrathoracic vessels. Thymic hypoplasia is seen in DiGeorge syndrome in association with aortic arch anomalies, immune and parathyroid dysfunction, and absence of the thymus can usually be confirmed in suspected cases by ultrasound in infancy.

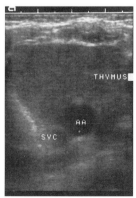

(b)

The normal thymus has homogenous echogenicity. SVC: superior vena cava; AA: ascending aorta.

Adam, E. J. and Ignotus, P. I. (1993). Sonography of the thymus in healthy children: frequency of visualization, size and appearance. *Am. J. Roentgenol.*, **161**, 153–5.

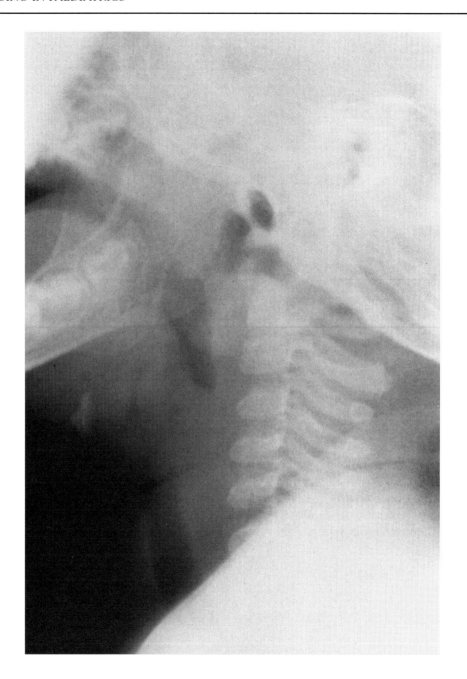

What abnormality is evident on the lateral neck radiograph in this child with fever and drooling?

Epiglottitis

The epiglottis is enlarged and protrudes posteriorly into the pharyngeal airspace. There is also marked swelling of the aryepiglottic folds.

Epiglottitis, caused by infection with *Haemophilus influenzae* type b, occurs predominantly in preschool age children. The onset is acute with inspiratory stridor, fever, drooling, and signs of systemic toxicity. Fatal airway obstruction can occur within hours. The aryepiglottic folds are thin bands of tissue connecting the epiglottis to the upper oesophageal region and when enlarged in acute epiglottitis account for much of the airway obstruction.

Radiology is unnecessary when the diagnosis of epiglottitis is clear. If a child with suspected epiglottitis is so well as to cast doubt on the diagnosis then a lateral neck radiograph may be justifiable. Although the role of radiology in the diagnosis of epiglottitis is controversial, recognition of a swollen epiglottis is of paramount importance. When radiographs are performed in doubtful cases the appropriate equipment and personnel skilled in the management of the pediatric airway should be in attendance at all times.

Other causes of airway obstruction to consider in the differential diagnosis include croup (laryngotracheitis), bacterial tracheitis, impacted foreign body, and retropharyngeal abscess. In croup, the primary abnormality on X-ray is subglottic oedema with ill-defined narrowing of the subglottis; the epiglottis and aryepiglottic folds are normal. With epiglottitis, the epiglottis and aryepiglottic folds are markedly enlarged though some mild subglottic oedema can also be evident. On the lateral neck radiograph of the child with acute epiglottitis the pharynx is often distended with air due to the airway obstruction and the neck is typically held in extension.

Cressman, W. R. and Myer, C. M. (1994). Diagnosis and management of croup and epiglottitis. *Pediatr. Clin. North Am.*, **41**, 265–76.

McCook, T. A. and Kirks, D. R. (1982). Epiglottic enlargement in infants and children: another radiologic look. *Pediatr. Radiol.*, **12**, 227–34.

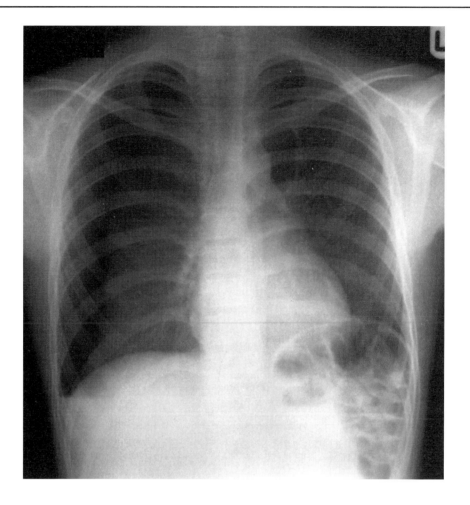

What is the cause of this teenager's chest pain?

Right pneumothorax

The right hemithorax is larger than the left with some flattening of the right hemidiaphragm. A free lung edge, typical of a pneumothorax, is visible in the right chest with no lung markings evident in the periphery of the hemithorax.

After the neonatal period, spontaneous pneumothorax is uncommon in the young child but not infrequent in adolescence. Pleuritic pain rather than dyspnoea is the usual predominant clinical feature in older children. A pneumothorax is a relatively common complication of cystic fibrosis, but pneumomediastinum rather than pneumothorax is a more common association in childhood asthma. Although an expiratory radiograph can make visualization of a small pneumothorax easier, smaller pneumothoraces are usually not clinically significant making such a procedure rarely necessary.

A pneumothorax is probably more frequent in the newborn period than at any other time in childhood, and is commonly related to intubation or resuscitation, meconium aspiration syndrome, or hyaline membrane disease. In neonates and infants, particular care must be taken to differentiate an axillary skin fold from a loculated pneumothorax. Small pneumothoraces can be difficult to detect in babies and younger children who routinely have radiographs taken in the supine position. In these supine patients free air tends to locate anteriorly and medially at the anterior cardiophrenic angles often causing an asymmetric, clearly defined cardiac border on the side of the pneumothorax, due to the free air, rather than aerated lung, being directly adjacent to the heart shadow.

Moskowitz, P. S. and Thorne Griscom, N. (1976). The medial pneumothorax. *Radiology*, **120**, 143–7.

Mayo, P. and Saha, S. P. (1983). Spontaneous pneumothorax in the newborn. *Am. Surg.*, **49**, 192–5.

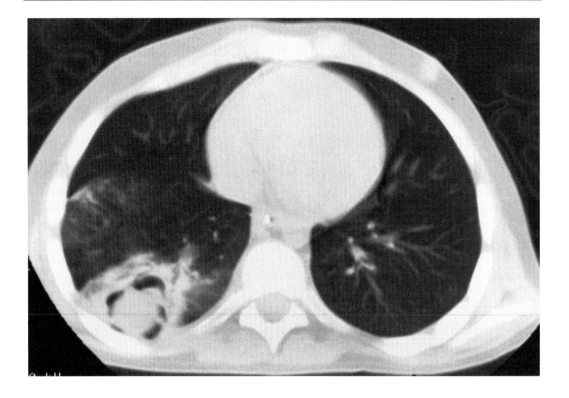

What lesion is evident on CT in an immunocompromised child on anti-leukaemic chemotherapy?

Mycetoma (aspergilloma)

There is a rounded opacity due to a fungus ball or mycetoma within a large cavity in the right lower lobe with adjacent parenchymal consolidation. A small amount of pleural thickening is present medial to the lesion.

Focal invasive pulmonary aspergillosis can develop rapidly in the debilitated or immunocompromised host, such as children on chemotherapy, with subsequent cavitation and the development of an intracavitary mass. A mycetoma is an intracavitary conglomeration of fungal hyphae matted together with fibrin, mucous, and cellular debris. When known to be caused by aspergillus species, the term aspergilloma is used synonymously. Productive cough is usual and frequently accompanied by haemoptysis which can be copious with a risk of fatal exsanguination.

Radiologically, fungus balls can initially be indistinguishable from a simple area of consolidation but with progressive cavitation the rounded shadowing will become separated from the wall of the cavity by an airspace of variable size giving the easily recognizable 'crescent sign' of a fungus ball in a pulmonary cavity. Intracavitary fungus balls are more common in the upper lobes in debilitated patients and often have associated pleural thickening with occasional periosteal reaction along adjacent ribs. Plain radiographs are usually diagnostic but CT can be confirmatory in doubtful cases.

Bomelburg, T., Roos, N., von Lengerke, H. J., and Ritter, J. (1992). Invasive aspergillosis complicating induction chemotherapy of childhood leukaemia. *Eur. J. Pediatr.*, **151**, 485–7.

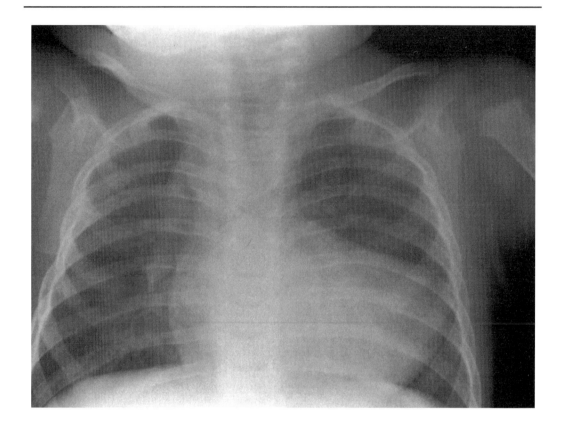

This child was noted to be cyanotic at three months of age. What is the diagnosis? Describe the radiographic findings.

Tetralogy of Fallot

There is elevation of the cardiac apex due to right ventricular enlargement. The pulmonary trunk region (left upper cardiac border) is under-developed giving a characteristic boot-shaped cardiac shadow. Pulmonary vascularity is reduced particularly in the left lung. The aortic arch is right sided and deformity of the right fourth and fifth ribs is due to a previous thoracotomy for a Blalock shunt.

Tetralogy of Fallot is the commonest congenital cyanotic heart disease. It comprises:

(1) ventricular septal defect (VSD)

(2) infundibular pulmonary stenosis

(3) an aorta that overrides the ventricular septum

(4) right ventricular hypertrophy.

A right aortic arch occurs in 25% of cases and is recognizable on chest radiographs as an indentation on the right side of the trachea with absence of the normal left sided aortic knuckle and descending aorta. The pulmonary vasculature may be oligaemic or normal but accurate estimation of pulmonary vascularity is very difficult on plain radiographs. The heart size is usually normal. The radiographic appearances are often diagnostic in tetralogy of Fallot but echocardiography is necessary to confirm an enlarged aortic root overriding a VSD, pulmonary stenosis, and right ventricular hypertrophy.

Armstrong, B. E. (1995). Congenital cardiovascular disease and cardiac surgery in childhood. Part I. Cyanotic congenital heart defects. *Curr. Opin. Cardiol.*, **10**, 58–67.

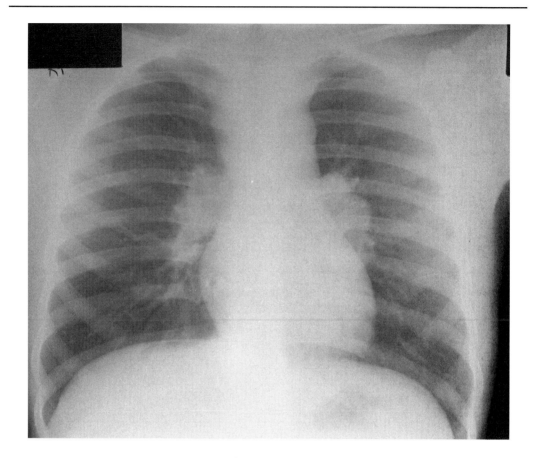

List two abnormalities present on the chest radiograph. What is the most likely diagnosis?

1. Hilar adenopathy
2. Mediastinal adenopathy
3. Lymphoma (non-Hodgkin's)

There is lobular shadowing in both hila, distinct from the vascular markings, typical of hilar adenopathy. In addition, the superior mediastinum is widened secondary to adenopathy. The lungs are clear.

Non-Hodgkin's lymphoma (NHL) accounts for 60% of childhood lymphomas. NHL comprises a heterogenous group of lymphoproliferative disorders of T-cell or B-cell lineage (including Burkitt's lymphoma), plus histiocytic and mixed cell types. T-cell lymphoma accounts for approximately 35% of NHL cases and generally presents with intrathoracic lymphadenopathy with or without lung parenchymal involvement. Pleural, pericardial, and lung involvement are more common in NHL than in Hodgkin's disease. Superior vena caval obstruction or tracheal compression may occur in both types of lymphoma but tend to be more severe in NHL. Staging is based on clinical examination, haematological investigations and an evaluation of the extent of the disease, best assessed by imaging.

Lymphoma can have variable radiographic manifestations ranging from a solitary nodule to bulky masses of tumour. Pleural or pericardial effusions are relatively common with NHL. Chest and abdominal CT, or MRI when feasible, are routinely performed for staging purposes at diagnosis and intermittently during follow-up to monitor response to treatment. Renal ultrasound is usually performed also at presentation to exclude renal lymphoma or obstruction secondary to nodal masses. Imaging of the central nervous system is reserved for patients with symptoms or signs of CNS disease. Radionuclide Gallium 67 citrate scanning is occasionally useful in searching for small amounts of disease activity during follow-up.

The differential diagnosis of bilateral hilar adenopathy in children also includes viral infections, sarcoidosis, cyclosporin related lymphoproliferative disease, and tuberculosis though the latter is rarely bilateral or symmetrical.

Carty, H. and Martin, J. (1993). Staging of lymphoma in childhood. *Clin. Radiol.*, **48**, 151–9.

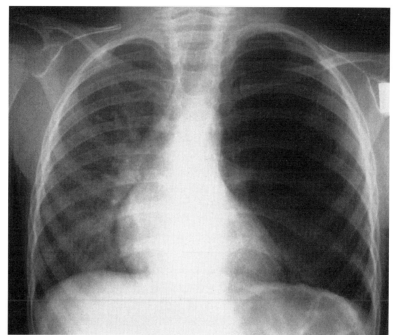

(a)

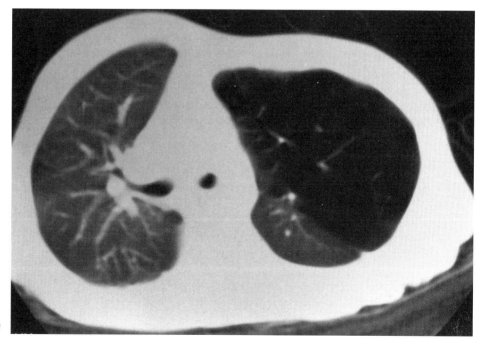

(b)

Chest radiograph and CT in a two year old with mild but stable respiratory symptoms. What is the diagnosis?

Congenital lobar emphysema

The mediastinum is shifted to the right with increased transradiancy and reduced vascularity in the left hemithorax. Vascular 'markings' are faintly visible in the periphery of the lung and there is no evidence of a lung edge to suggest a pneumothorax. The CT shows a normal right lung with overinflation and emphysema of the left upper lobe and compression of a normal left lower lobe.

Congenital lobar emphysema, or simply lobar emphysema as some cases may be acquired, is an important cause of respiratory distress in children. In the newborn period lobar emphysema can present with severe respiratory distress, but in infancy and later childhood, symptoms may be mild and intermittent. In general, the earlier the presentation the more severe the symptoms and the greater likelihood that surgical removal of the overinflated lobe will be necessary. The left upper lobe, right middle lobe and right upper lobe are affected in order of decreasing frequency. Mild cases in older children are now usually managed conservatively. Congenital heart disease e.g. absent pulmonary valves is found in up to 20% of infants with lobar emphysema.

Overdistension of a single lobe with increased transradiancy, oligaemia, and mediastinal shift are the usual radiographic findings. Prolonged retention of foetal lung fluid can initially obscure the emphysematous lobe in neonates causing a transient lobar mass or consolidation until the fluid clears and is replaced by air. Compression atelectasis of uninvolved adjacent lobes can often be best appreciated on CT scanning. CT is also useful in order to exclude an extrinsic mass such as a mediastinal bronchogenic cyst leading to obstructive emphysema but such mass lesions usually result in whole lung, rather than lobar, emphysema. Ventilation-perfusion lung scans can show poor perfusion and reduced ventilation of the affected lobe but plain radiographs supplemented by CT are usually sufficient to make the diagnosis.

Cleveland, R. H. and Weber, B. (1993). Retained fetal lung liquid in congenital lobar emphysema: a possible predictor of polyalveolar lobe. *Pediatr. Radiol.*, **23**, 291–5.

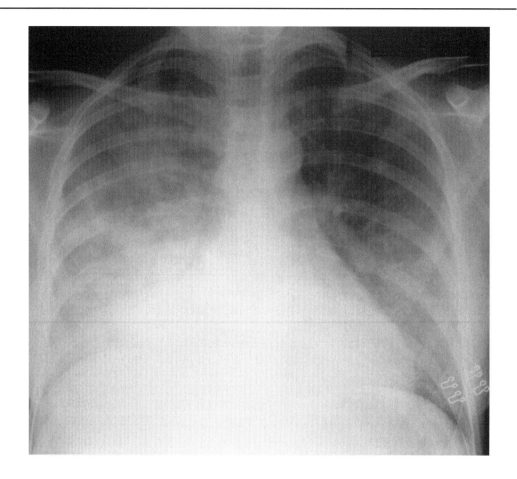

This adolescent female had an episode of near drowning. The chest radiograph was taken six days later. What complication has occurred?

Adult respiratory distress syndrome (ARDS)

There is confluent air-space consolidation bilaterally resulting in virtually complete white-out of both lungs, but with some sparing of the left upper zone.

A normal chest radiograph on admission in the setting of near drowning has a good prognosis. Duration of submersion, water temperature, and concomitant cerebral injury all have a significant influence on the chest radiographic findings and clinical outcome. Salinity of the water is thought to be less important than temperature, with cold water injury having a better outlook. Lung changes usually resolve within a week unless there is superadded pneumonia or ARDS.

Lung 'white-out' from diffuse consolidation has numerous causes. Simplistically, widespread fluid due to oedema, pulmonary haemorrhage, pus, or combinations of these can all result in diffuse parenchymal opacities. Pulmonary oedema secondary to cardiac decompensation is typically accompanied by cardiomegaly, whilst in non-cardiogenic pulmonary oedema cardiac enlargement does not occur. Other recognized causes of diffuse air-space shadowing include smoke inhalation, pulmonary aspiration, and lipid pneumonia. ARDS, which manifests as widespread air-space consolidation usually in the setting of multiorgan failure, has a high mortality. Although the radiographic features of many of the above conditions are similar, the clinical history and course of the patient will usually indicate the correct aetiology.

Levin, D. L., Morriss, F. C., Toro, L. O. *et al.* (1993). Drowning and near-drowning. *Pediatr. Clin. North Am.*, **40**, 321–6.

Effman, E. L., Merton, D. F., Kirks, D. R. *et al.* (1985). Adult respiratory distress syndrome in children. *Radiology*, **157**, 69–74.

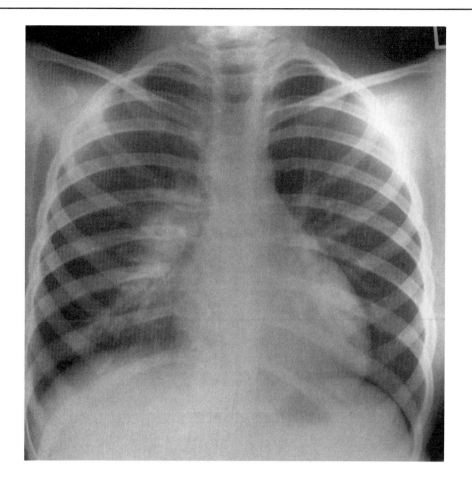

This child had anorexia, weight loss, and a low-grade fever. What is the likely diagnosis?

Primary tuberculosis

There is a small parenchymal nodule or shadowing in the right lower zone with associated enlargement of the right hilar lymph nodes.

Primary tuberculosis is the disease produced by a first infection with tubercle bacilli, and includes the primary complex and subsequent progression of the primary infection. The primary or Ghon complex refers to a parenchymal lesion with associated regional adenopathy. A pleural effusion may be seen in association with the primary complex but is relatively uncommon in children less than six years. Primary tuberculosis is usually innocuous with healing and calcification of the Ghon complex often occurring within 12 months.

Enlarged mediastinal lymph nodes can, however, compress the adjacent bronchi leading to incomplete obstruction with either distal hyperinflation or lobar collapse. Caseating lymph nodes may occasionally erode through a bronchus resulting in tuberculous bronchopneumonia. Younger children are particularly susceptible to miliary tuberculosis resulting from haematogenous dissemination of tubercle bacilli. Miliary tuberculosis may occur up to one year after an untreated primary tuberculous lesion and manifests on chest radiographs as fine nodular shadowing in both lungs often without associated adenopathy.

Strouse, P. J., Dessner, D. A., Watson, W. J., and Blane, C. E. (1996). Mycobacterium tuberculosis infection in immunocompetent children. *Pediatr. Radiol.*, **26**, 134–40.

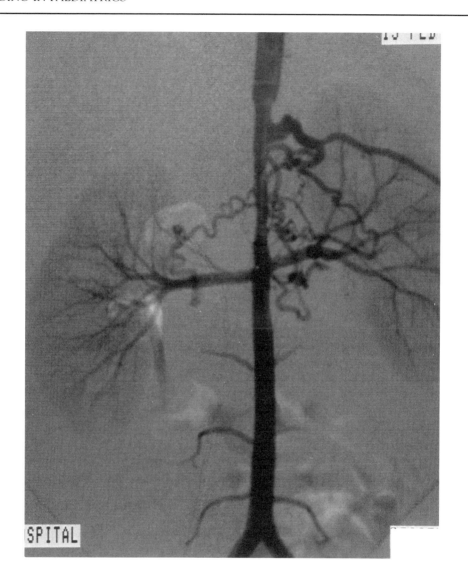

What is the abnormality on the abdominal aortogram in this adolescent with hypertension?

Middle aortic syndrome

This digital subtraction angiogram shows irregular narrowing of the lower thoracic and upper abdominal aorta. Other oblique images also revealed narrowing at the origins of both renal arteries. A few tortuous retroperitoneal vessels are present, and there is no opacification of the vessels of the coeliac trunk, superior or inferior mesenteric arteries indicating complete occlusion.

Middle aortic syndrome is defined by the angiographic findings of tubular stenosis of the abdominal aorta in the absence of any clinical or biochemical evidence of arteritis. Unlike Takayasu's arteritis, middle aortic syndrome tends to arrest at puberty; there is no fever, myalgia, or elevation of the ESR and no pulmonary artery involvement. Involvement of the renal arteries leading to hypertension is a frequent complication. Surgery is usually recommended only after medical anti-hypertensive treatment has failed. Involvement of the mesenteric vessels is also a relatively frequent angiographic finding in middle aortic syndrome but mesenteric angina is uncommon due to hypertrophied collaterals.

Robinson, L., Gedroyc, W., Reidy, J., and Saxton, H. M. (1991). Renal artery stenosis in children. *Clin. Radiol.*, **44**, 376–82.

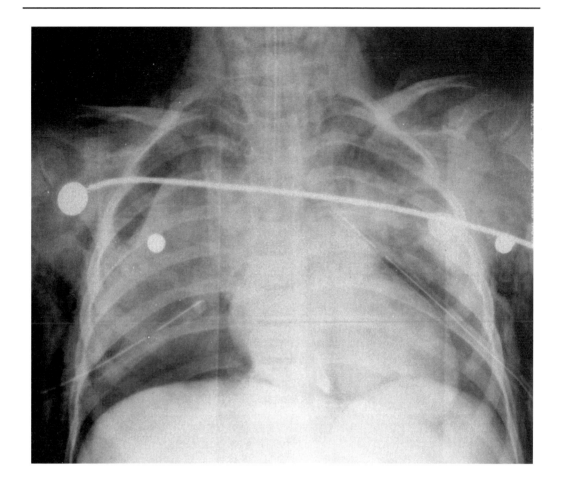

This young child has been injured in a road traffic accident. List four abnormalities on the chest radiograph.

1. Subcutaneous emphysema
2. Right pneumothorax
3. Pulmonary contusions
4. A tooth is visible in the distal oesophagus

The chest X-ray was taken as a portable emergency film. Chest drains have been inserted for bilateral pneumothoraces. The right-sided pneumothorax persisted for a number of days and was eventually found to be secondary to a partial tear of the right main bronchus. Shadowing in both lungs in the context of severe trauma is likely due to pulmonary contusion and the tooth may have been dislodged during emergency intubation. No rib fractures are visible. Linear artefacts are due to a trauma board.

Chest trauma can result in injury to the bony skeleton, mediastinal vascular structures, or lungs with a variety of radiologic manifestations. Subcutaneous crepitus on palpation should alert the clinician to the presence of subcutaneous emphysema and the possibility of an underlying air-leak. Furthermore, persistent leakage of air into the pleura or mediastinum despite adequately placed intercostal drains increases the likelihood of a traumatic broncho-pleural fistula or even major tracheobronchial rupture, which would require surgical repair. Associated rib fractures may be evident but fractures of the thoracic cage can be extremely difficult to identify on initial chest films and may only become visible some days later when healing callus begins to form.

Pulmonary contusion secondary to blunt chest trauma can cause a variety of radiographic changes ranging from patchy shadowing to widespread consolidation. These changes are generally visible within hours after the episode of trauma. Localized haematomas can occasionally cavitate or be complicated by superadded infection.

Roux, P. and Fisher, R. M. (1992). Chest injuries in children: an analysis of 100 cases of blunt chest trauma from motor vehicle accidents. *J. Pediatr. Surg.*, **27**, 551–5.

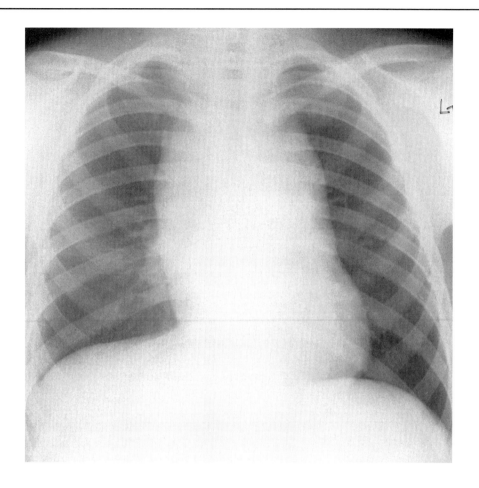

This is the chest radiograph of a child with widespread adenopathy and a haemoglobin of 6 g/dl. What is the diagnosis?

Mediastinal mass: secondary to leukaemia

There is widening of the superior mediastinum with loss of visualization of the normal contours of the aortic knuckle and pulmonary trunk, due to a conglomerate nodal mass lesion overlying these structures.

A mediastinal mass is evident at presentation in approximately 15% of children with acute lymphoblastic leukaemia (usually T-cell leukaemia).

The interface between a smooth soft tissue outline such as the cardiac shadow and air in the lungs gives a clear margin provided the interface is tangential to the X-ray beam. When an opacity or mass replaces the air, the radiographic boundary is lost. The *silhouette sign* refers to loss of the normal silhouette of any of the usual cardiac borders. Loss of the silhouette of the pulmonary trunk, aortic arch, and aortic knuckle in the illustration indicate that the conglomerate mass is predominantly in the middle mediastinum, immediately adjacent to these structures.

Gomez, E., San Miguel, J. F., Gonzalez, M., *et al.* (1991). Heterogeneity of T-cell lymphoblastic leukaemias. *J. Clin. Pathol.*, **44**, 628–31.

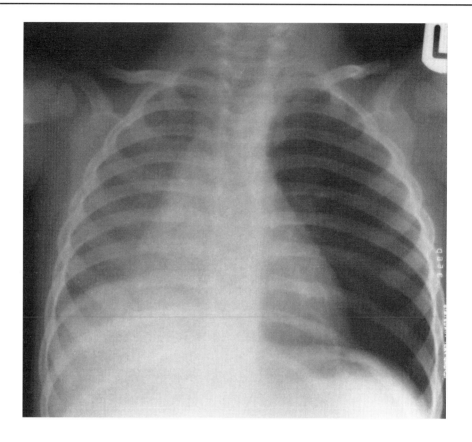

What is the most likely explanation for the abnormality on this expiratory chest radiograph?

Inhaled foreign body

There is air-trapping with overinflation of the left lung due to partial obstruction of the left main bronchus by an aspirated foreign body. Normal reduction in volume with expiration has occurred on the right side.

The majority of inhaled foreign bodies are non-opaque, and the most frequently aspirated items are vegetable matter or small nuts, particularly peanuts. A history of sudden choking with acute onset of respiratory distress may be obtained but symptoms can be delayed with later cough, wheezing, or haemoptysis. The radiographic findings depend on the size, duration, location, and nature of the inhaled foreign body.

Whenever an aspirated foreign body is suspected, expiratory radiographs should be performed because in the acute phase standard (inspiratory) chest radiographs may appear normal, with air-trapping or obstructive emphysema becoming evident only on expiration. Lung overinflation results in a flat hemidiaphragm, widened rib spaces, attenuated pulmonary vessels, and mediastinal deviation away from the side of the abnormality. An air-leak with a pneumomediastinum or pneumothorax may be associated. Although CT is more sensitive than plain radiography in the detection of aspirated foreign bodies, bronchoscopy is the definitive diagnostic and therapeutic manoeuvre and is generally considered a better alternative. Undiagnosed aspiration may result in recurrent pneumonia, lobar collapse, or bronchiectasis.

Svedstrom, E., Puhakka, H., and Kero, P. (1989). How accurate is chest radiography in the diagnosis of tracheobronchial foreign bodies in children. *Pediatr. Radiol.*, **19**, 520–2.

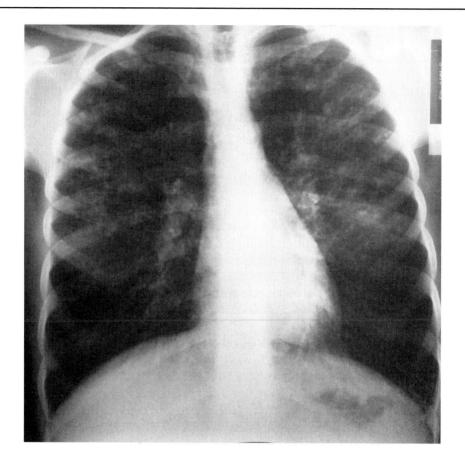

List three abnormalities on the chest radiograph in this child with recurrent respiratory infections and chronic cough. What is the diagnosis?

1. *Lung overinflation*
2. *Widespread peribronchial thickening*
3. *Bronchiectasis*

Cystic fibrosis

Lung hyperinflation manifests as low, flat hemidiaphragms and an increased anteroposterior diameter of the chest on lateral radiographs. Dilated thick-walled bronchi, particularly in the upper zones, reflect diffuse bronchiectasis.

Cystic fibrosis is an inherited autosomal recessive disease, with the highest incidence of approximately 1 in 2500 live births occurring in Caucasian families of European background. Pancreatic insufficiency and chronic suppurative lung disease are the major manifestations. Infections with *Staphylococcus aureus* and pseudomonas species are frequent. Less commonly, bronchopulmonary aspergillosis leading to widespread areas of consolidation which clear and recur rapidly can cause severe parenchymal destruction. Acute deterioration due to a pneumothorax is a well-recognized association.

Accentuation of the bronchial wall pattern with peribronchial thickening, and bronchiectasis manifesting as parallel line ('tram-line') and ring shadows are typical features on chest radiographs. Segmental bronchiectasis tends to affect the upper lobes more frequently but all lobes can be affected. Prominence of the hila is often seen due either to lymph node enlargement or pulmonary artery dilatation with concomitant pulmonary hypertension. Several methods for scoring the severity of the lung changes in cystic fibrosis exist but are subject to much inter-observer variability and pulmonary function testing with clinical evaluation remain the cornerstone of lung disease assessment.

Mukhopadhay, S., Kirby, M. L., Duncan, A. W., and Carswell, F. (1996). Early focal abnormalities on chest radiographs and respiratory prognosis in children with cystic fibrosis. *Br. J. Radiol.*, **69**, 122–5.

Shale, D. J. (1994). Chest radiology in cystic fibrosis: is scoring useful? *Thorax*, **49**, 847.

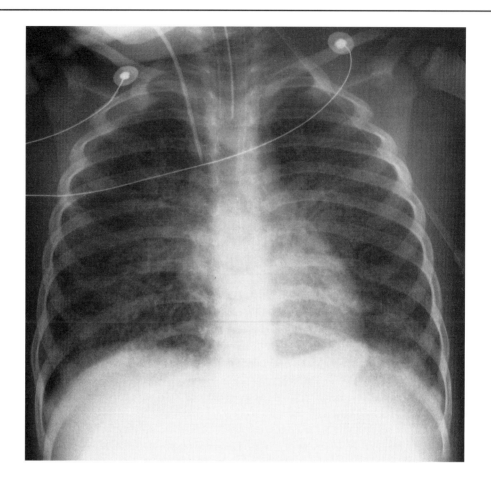

This child presented with fever and tachypnoea, with deteriorating blood gases necessitating mechanical ventilation. What is the most likely aetiology?

Viral pneumonia

There is bilateral reticular, interstitial shadowing mainly in a perihilar and lower zone distribution. Prominence of the hila bilaterally suggest some additional hilar adenopathy. A small right apical pleural effusion is present. The central venous line, ET and NG tubes are correctly sited (the tip of the NG tube was clearly visible in the stomach on the better penetrated original radiograph). The heart size is normal.

Bacterial pulmonary infection generally manifests as confluent lobar opacification. Reticular or linear shadowing in the pulmonary interstitium is commonly due to either cardiac failure or viral infection. A normal heart size makes cardiogenic pulmonary oedema unlikely.

The radiographic features of viral pneumonia are variable and non-specific. Viral infection commonly manifests with bronchial wall thickening, peribronchial densities, air trapping, and patchy or confluent infiltrates. Nevertheless, reticular (linear) shadowing in the interstitium is a well-recognized radiographic appearance of viral lower respiratory tract infection. Causative agents include adenovirus, influenza, parainfluenza, and respiratory syncytial virus (RSV). In addition to these, cytomegalovirus, measles, and varicella can also result in severe interstitial pneumonia in immunocompromised children. However, RSV more commonly gives rise to a 'bronchiolitis pattern' i.e. widespread peribronchial thickening with patchy atelectasis and air trapping.

A variety of other pathologies can manifest in children as an interstitial lung process. *Chlamydia trachomatis* in early infancy and *Mycoplasma* infection in later childhood are two recognized non-viral, infectious causes of interstitial lung shadowing. *Pneumocystic carinii* pneumonia in the immunosuppressed host, and lymphocytic interstitial pneumonitis (LIP) in children with AIDS, are two other important causes of interstitial shadowing.

Wildin, S. R., Chonmaitree, T., and Swischuk, L. E. (1988). Roentgenographic features of common pediatric viral respiratory tract infections. *Am. J. Dis. Child.*, **142**, 43–6.

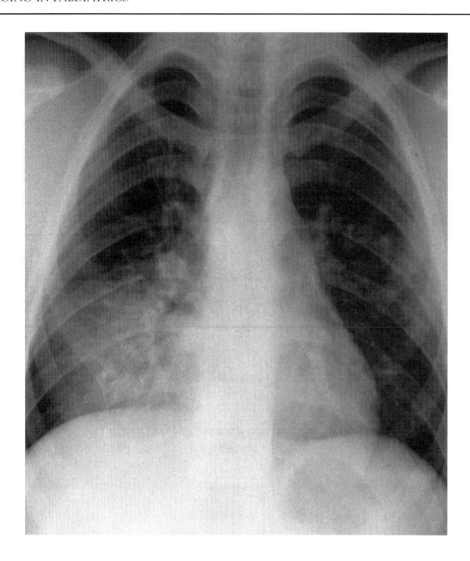

What is the cause of this child's fever and tachypnoea?

Right middle lobe pneumonia

There is confluent consolidation in the lower zone of the right lung with loss of the right cardiac silhouette characteristic of right middle lobe pneumonia. Note the outline of the right hemidiaphragm is preserved indicating a normally aerated right lower lobe.

The medial aspect of the right middle lobe abuts the right cardiac border. Loss of the right cardiac silhouette localizes consolidation to the right middle lobe. Consolidation in the lingula results in a similar loss of the left cardiac silhouette; pneumonia in the basal segments of the lower lobes leads to an obscured ipsilateral hemidiaphragm.

On a chest radiograph, lobar or segmental pneumonia manifests as confluent, homogenous opacification often with an air bronchogram. Bacterial infection e.g. pneumococcal pneumonia classically results in lobar consolidation. Many bacterial pathogens cause identical radiographic appearances but pneumatoceles i.e. thin-walled, air-containing cavities, usually result from staphylococcal infection. Prior to the introduction of the Hib vaccine, *Haemophilus influenzae* was a frequent cause of pulmonary consolidation in children less than two years of age.

Mycoplasma pneumoniae is the most common single cause of pneumonia in childhood and has a variable radiographic appearance ranging from a reticular, interstitial pattern to confluent, bilateral air-space consolidation. The chest radiographic appearances in *Mycoplasma* infection are characteristically more widespread and impressive than the patient's clinical condition.

With simple lobar consolidation follow-up radiography is not required after good clinical response to treatment. When there has been lobar collapse, segmental consolidation, or poor response to treatment, follow-up chest radiographs are essential to rule out an underlying treatable process e.g. aspirated foreign body.

Korrpi, M., Kiekara, O., Heiskanen-Kosma, T., and Soimakallio, S. (1993). Comparison of radiological findings and microbial aetiology of childhood pneumonia. *Acta. Pediatr.*, **82**, 360–3.

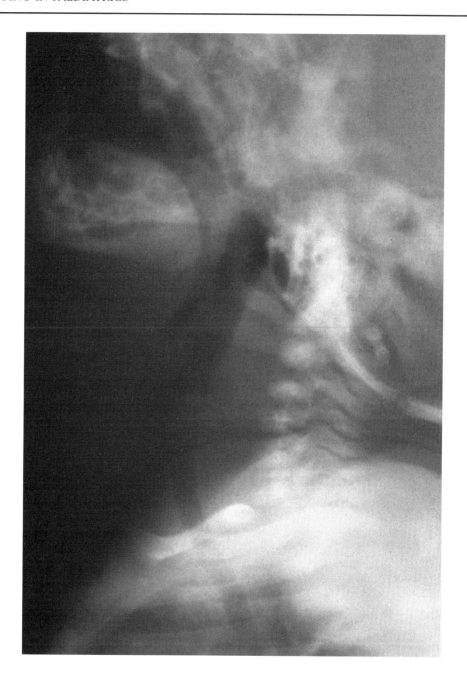

What abnormality is present on the lateral neck radiograph in this child with fever, drooling, and torticollis?

Retropharyngeal abscess

There is marked pre-vertebral soft tissue swelling with forward displacement of the hypopharynx and airway. This swelling could be due to either a retropharyngeal haematoma or abscess/infection, but in the clinical context infection is likely.

The retropharyngeal lymph nodes tend to atrophy around three to five years of age such that a retropharyngeal abscess due to suppuration in these nodes generally occurs in early childhood. Retropharyngeal nodes receive drainage from the middle ear, tonsils and pharynx, all of which are common sites of childhood infection. A staphylococcal or streptococcal organism is generally responsible. Pharyngeal perforation resulting in a retropharyngeal abscess can occur secondary to a penetrating injury from a swallowed sharp foreign body or can be secondary to intubation. Child abuse is another recognized cause of pharyngeal perforation and retropharyngeal infection. Dysphagia is frequently present and mediastinitis can ensue.

A lateral neck film is obtained during inspiration with the neck partially extended. Expiration, swallowing, and neck flexion during exposure of the radiograph can all cause confusing bulging of the pliant soft tissues of a child's neck. If doubt exists regarding the validity of the findings, then the radiograph should be repeated taking care to ensure exposure during inspiration. The hyoid is normally situated a few centimetres inferior to the mandible and swallowing can often be recognized on a radiograph by elevation of the hyoid to a level at or above the angle of the mandible. The normal pre-vertebral space in the lower cervical region should be no wider than the A–P diameter of a vertebral body. A retropharyngeal haematoma or infection can be identical on plain radiographs but air in a retropharyngeal collection is diagnostic of an abscess. In the context of an abscess, CT is occasionally helpful by its ability to quantify accurately the amount of purulent material prior to drainage.

Swischuk, L. E. (1995). Stiff neck with fever. *Pediatr. Emerg. Care.*, **11**, 199–200.

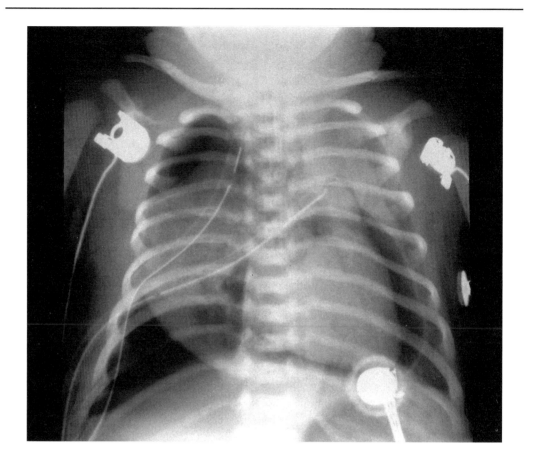

This is a post-operative chest radiograph of an infant who had surgery for removal of a congenital cystic adenomatoid malformation (CCAM) in the right lung. List three abnormalities.

1. *Right pneumothorax*
2. *Pneumopericardium—from excessive medial placement of the lower chest drain*
3. *Lucencies in partially collapsed right lung due to residual CCAM*

CCAM usually involves only one lobe of a lung but occasionally multiple lobes are involved. Perioperative complications precluded initial complete resection in the above case.

A pneumopericardium manifests on a chest film as a lucent halo around the heart due to air in the pericardial sac. Common causes of a pneumopericardium include mechanical ventilation in the newborn, asthma, trauma, and surgery. A pneumopericardium may be difficult to differentiate from a pneumomediastinum. Air inferior to the heart separating the cardiac shadow from the central tendon of the diaphragm, in addition to a clearly outlined pericardial sac, help distinguish a pneumopericardium from a pneumomediastinum. With a pneumopericardium the main pulmonary artery may be outlined by pericardial air and air does not rise to the level of the aortic arch which is outside the pericardial cavity. In a pneumomediastinum, the free air in the mediastinum usually extends superiorly above the cardiac shadow and can also elevate the thymus making it more clearly visible leading to a characteristic sail-shaped shadow.

Van Gelderen, W. F. (1993). Stab wounds of the heart: two new signs of pneumopericardium. *Br. J. Radiol.*, **66**, 794–6.

.

3. Gastrointestinal and genitourinary

Splenic haematoma

Appendicitis

Vesicoureteric reflux

Small bowel obstruction secondary to hernia

Meckel's diverticulum

Sacral agenesis

Posterior urethral valves

Adrenal calcification

Hypertrophic pyloric stenosis

Pneumoperitoneum

Colonopathy in cystic fibrosis

Hydronephrosis

Crohn's disease

Wilms' tumour

Biliary atresia

Trichobezoar

Intussusception

Duplex kidney

Neuroblastoma

Renal scarring

Urachal cyst abscess

Pelvi-ureteric junction obstruction

Caustic oesophagitis

Choledochal cyst

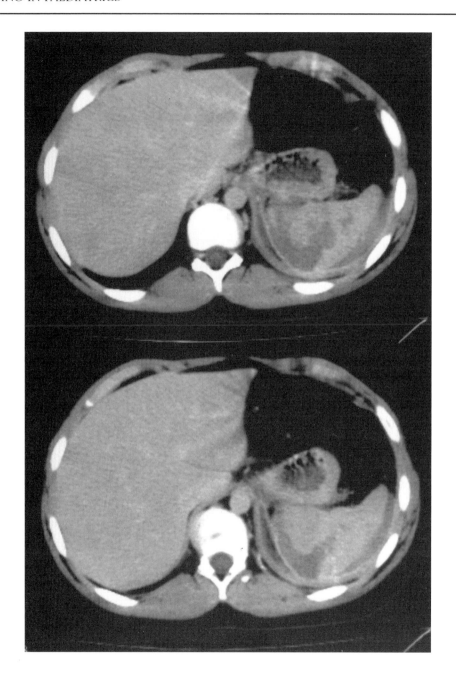

What abnormality is evident on the contiguous CT sections in this boy who was injured in a road traffic accident?

Splenic haematoma

There is heterogeneous low attenuation throughout much of the spleen in keeping with a splenic haematoma. Perisplenic fluid (blood) is seen surrounding the posterior aspect of the spleen.

Blunt trauma can result in injury to any abdominal viscus and the spleen is particularly susceptible. Splenic injuries range from small subcapsular haematomas, to more extensive parenchymal haematomas, lacerations, or complete fracture of the splenic body, often with an associated haemoperitoneum. There has been an increasing trend in recent years towards non-operative management of splenic trauma in the haemodynamically stable patient, mainly because of the increased risk of sepsis following splenectomy. The size of a splenic injury should not determine management and the decision to operate is based primarily on the clinical condition of the child.

Where CT is available it is generally superior to ultrasound in the evaluation of blunt abdominal trauma as a comprehensive examination of the entire abdominal contents is possible. Perisplenic fluid or a haemoperitoneum are commonly found in association with a splenic injury. Other possible causes of free intra-abdominal fluid may also be recognized e.g. renal, hepatic, or bowel injuries. However, CT cannot determine whether active splenic bleeding is taking place—a haemoperitoneum merely reflects the cumulative total of bleeding that occurred between the time of injury and the CT examination.

Ultrasound is favoured in some centres initially to assess the solid abdominal viscera in the setting of blunt trauma. However, assessment of the spleen can often be difficult due to overlying rib fractures. When free fluid or a solid organ injury are visible on ultrasound then it is generally advisable to perform a CT study to effect a complete abdominal examination.

Brick, S. H., Taylor, G. A., Potter, B. M., and Eichelberger, M. R. (1987). Hepatic and splenic injury in children: role of CT in the decision for laparotomy. *Radiology*, **165**, 643–6.

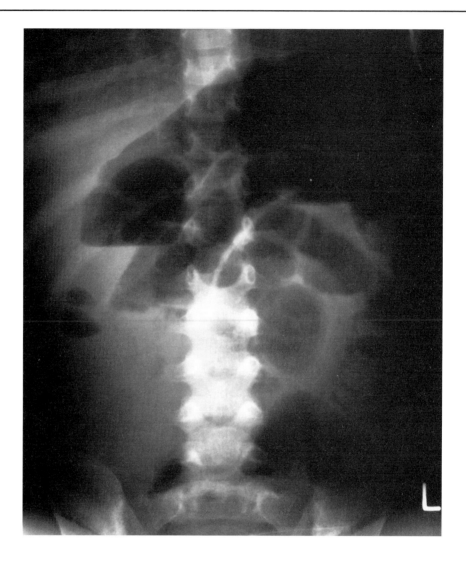

What abnormality is causing fever, vomiting, and abdominal pain in this four year old?

Appendicitis

A rounded density in the right iliac fossa due to a calcified faecolith in the appendix (appendicolith) is virtually diagnostic of appendicitis. There is a paucity of bowel gas in the right lower quadrant suggesting an associated inflammatory mass lesion. Gaseous distension of small and large bowel loops in the left and upper abdomen is caused by an ileus secondary to peritonitis.

Acute appendicitis is the most common indication for exploratory laparotomy in childhood and yet can be one of the most difficult diagnoses to make, particularly in younger children. Once suspected, the diagnosis is generally made on clinical grounds alone. Plain radiographs are usually normal in an uncomplicated case. A calcified faecolith inspissated in the appendix is visible in only 5–10% of children with appendicitis but when present in a suspected appendicitis confirms the diagnosis. However, an appendicolith may be located anywhere along the path of a retrocaecal appendix and can be mistaken for a renal calculus. Calcified appendicoliths are very occasionally picked up on plain films as an incidental finding. Elective appendicectomy at a later date is often performed in these circumstances.

Ultrasonography with graded compression to displace bowel gas from the right iliac fossa is a useful technique in doubtful cases in order to display the inflamed appendix and an associated inflammatory mass or abscess. An abscess collection can often be drained percutaneously under ultrasound guidance.

Sivit, C. J. (1993). Diagnosis of acute appendicitis in children: spectrum of sonographic findings. Am. J. Roentgenol., **161**, 147–52.

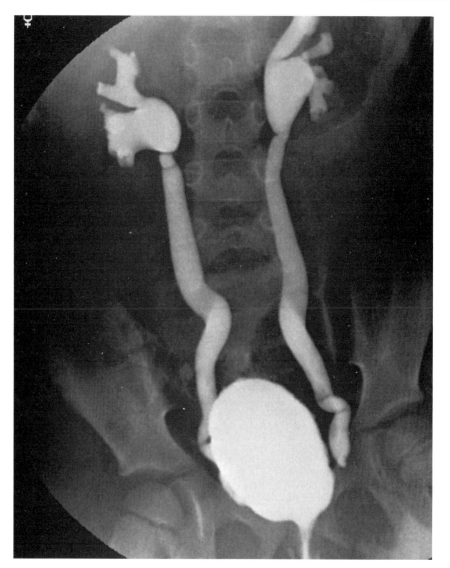

(a)

What abnormality is evident on this examination?

Bilateral vesicoureteric reflux (VUR)

The image in the illustration was taken during the voiding phase of a micturating or voiding cystourethrogram (MCUG or VCUG). Note contrast outlining the urethra inferior to the bladder base. There is reflux bilaterally into dilated ureters and renal collecting systems— grade III reflux.

The commonest indication for MCUG is as part of the investigation of young children with urinary tract infection. Other common indications include evaluation of antenatally diagnosed urinary tract abnormalities e.g. hydronephrosis or hydroureter, assessment of posterior urethral valves, neurogenic bladder, and in the evaluation of anorectal malformations to identify a recto-urinary fistula. A small (5–8F) feeding tube is inserted into the bladder via the urethra using an aseptic technique. A catheter without a balloon is preferred as an inflated balloon at the bladder neck runs the risk of completely obstructing the outlet leading to bladder rupture. Dilute contrast medium is instilled using a continuous infusion. The examination is terminated when the bladder has been filled and the patient has voided satisfactorily.

There is a small risk of urinary infection following catheterization and although strategies regarding antibiotic prophylaxis for MCUG vary, antibiotics are recommended in all patients in whom reflux is demonstrated. Conventional MCUG affords excellent anatomic information and is the recommended first imaging study in boys in whom detailed images of the urethra are necessary at the initial MCUG. As abnormalities of the female urethra are much less common, an isotope cystogram can be adequate as the first imaging study in girls. To reduce radiation and psychological trauma, direct radionuclide cystography or indirect MAG 3 cystography in toilet-trained children, are preferred for follow-up studies when feasible.

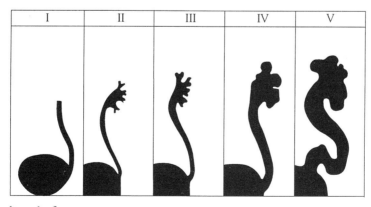

(b)

International grading of reflux.

Merrick, M. V., Notghi, A., Chalmers, N. *et al.* (1995). Long-term follow-up to determine the prognostic value of imaging after urinary tract infections. Part 1: reflux. *Arch. Dis. Child.*, **72**, 388–92.

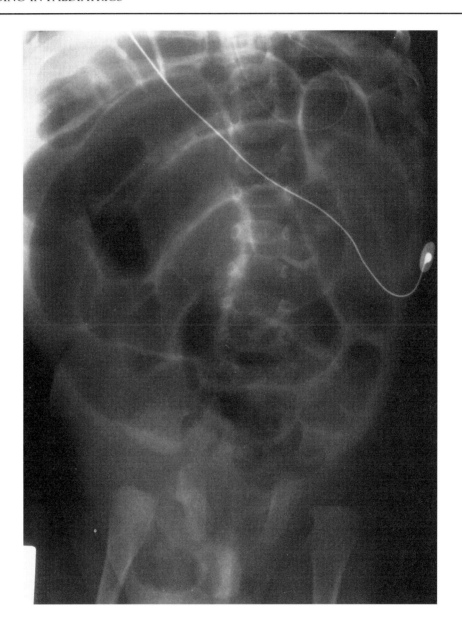

What abnormalities are evident on the plain abdominal radiograph in this male infant?

Small bowel obstruction due to a right inguinal hernia

There is gaseous distension of numerous small bowel loops throughout the abdomen with gas seen in the right side of the scrotum, and no bowel gas distally in the colon or rectum on a supine radiograph.

An incarcerated hernia is the commonest cause of intestinal obstruction in infants between one and six months who have not had neonatal surgery. It is much more frequent in boys, commonly on the right side. The diagnosis is usually obvious clinically but radiographs without gonadal protection are occasionally necessary to confirm the clinical suspicion. With prolonged incarceration the hernia may be fluid-filled and airless but there is usually thickening of the inguino-scrotal region on the affected side.

A mechanical small bowel obstruction typically shows dilated small bowel loops predominantly in the mid-abdomen and left upper quadrant. Air-fluid levels are visible on erect and decubitus but not supine radiographs. In general, the more dilated loops or fluid levels visible on erect films, then the more distal is the obstruction but it should be remembered that bowel loops filled only with fluid are virtually impossible to visualize on abdominal radiographs. Complete mucosal folds (valvulae conniventes) can help distinguish the small intestine from large bowel, where the haustral pattern of folds does not completely encircle the bowel.

Common causes of small bowel obstruction in children include intussusception, incarceration in a hernia, adhesions, appendicitis, and small bowel volvulus. On viewing the radiograph, free intraperitoneal air due to perforation, the presence of a mass lesion or air trapped in a hernial orifice, or an appendicolith should be sought. The clinical findings will dictate the need for further imaging studies e.g. an incarcerated hernia warrants immediate surgery, whereas a suspected malrotation with volvulus would generally be confirmed with a pre-operative contrast study to define the position of the duodeno-jejunal junction.

Davies, N., Najmaldin, A., and Burge, D. M. (1990). Irreducible inguinal hernia in children below two years of age. *Br. J. Surg.*, **77**, 1291–2.

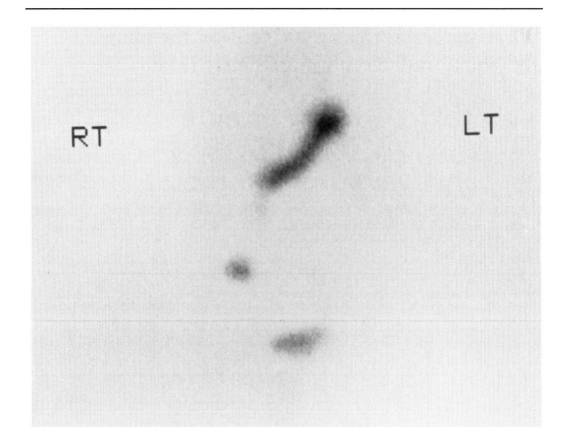

What lesion is evident in the abdomen on this radionuclide scan in a child with gastrointestinal bleeding?

Ectopic gastric mucosa in a Meckel's diverticulum

There is normal uptake of the radiopharmaceutical (technetium-99m pertechnetate) by the stomach. Some activity is also present in the bladder having been excreted by the kidneys and is a normal finding. Abnormal uptake of activity is seen to the right of the midline in the lower abdomen in ectopic gastric mucosa of a Meckel's diverticulum. The illustration was taken 60 minutes after injection of the radiopharmaceutical but it is important to remember that during a Meckel's study many dynamic images are taken in the search for simultaneous uptake of activity by the gastric mucosa of the stomach and by ectopic gastric mucosa.

Meckel's diverticulum occurs in approximately 2% of the population within 15 to 80 cm of the ileocaecal valve. A Meckel's diverticulum without gastric mucosa rarely bleeds. The 15% of Meckel's diverticula which do contain gastric mucosa can be complicated by peptic ulceration, perforation, and haemorrhage. Those diverticula that bleed generally present within the first 10 years of life with painless rectal haemorrhage and the diagnosis is usually confirmed by a standard Meckel's pertechnetate scan.

Diamond, R. H., Rothstein, R. D., and Aloni, A. (1991). Role of cimetidine-enhanced technetium-99m pertechnetate imaging for visualizing Meckel's diverticulum. *J. Nucl. Med.*, **32**, 1422–4.

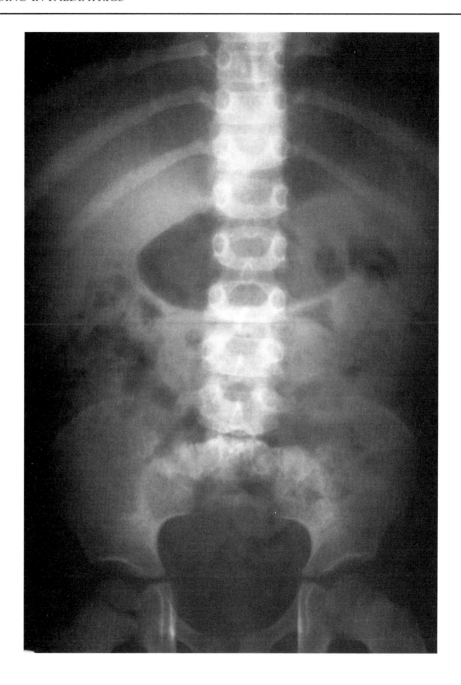

What is causing this child's urinary and faecal symptoms?

Sacral agenesis

The upper sacrum is hypoplastic with the iliac wings appearing somewhat closer together than is usual with complete absence of the lower sacral segments.

Milder degrees of sacral hypoplasia can pass unrecognized in the neonatal period and present in early childhood with problems in urinary and faecal continence. Constipation is a virtually constant feature of children with interruption of the normal neurogenic supply to bowel musculature, such as in spinal dysraphism or sacral agenesis. When assessing a plain abdominal radiograph in a child with constipation, careful attention should be paid to the development of the spine and sacrum as the treatment options and goals would be more limited in a child with underlying neurological impairment.

O'Neil, O. R., Piatt, J. H., Mitchell, P., and Roman-Goldstein, S. (1995). Agenesis and dysgenesis of the sacrum: neurosurgical implications. *Pediatr. Neurosurg.*, **22**, 20–8.

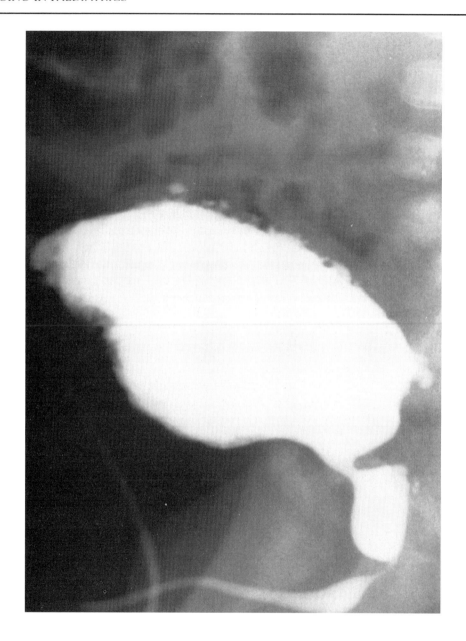

What abnormality is evident on this micturating cystourethrogram?

Posterior urethral valves

There is dilatation of the posterior urethra which is seen to terminate abruptly in a convex inferior border caused by obstructing valves. Bladder wall thickening and irregularity i.e. trabeculation is secondary to bladder outlet obstruction. A normal male anterior urethra is evident.

Posterior urethral valves occur exclusively in boys. The majority are actually unicuspid or bicuspid folds of mucosa at the level of verumontanum which result in obstruction to urinary flow. Formerly, presentation occurred secondary to a combination of a palpable bladder mass, urinary tract infection, or poor stream in a male infant. Posterior urethral valves are increasingly now suspected when antenatal ultrasound examinations reveal an enlarged posterior urethra, thick-walled bladder, or upper tract dilatation.

Bladder outlet obstruction tends to result in bilateral vesicoureteric reflux which in turn leads to hydronephrosis and renal dysplastic changes. The high pressure urinary system can be complicated by a caliceal leak of urine manifesting on ultrasound as a perinephric urinoma or urinary ascites. Decompression of the bladder via reflux into dilated ureters and via a caliceal leak can occasionally result in a small bladder. Postnatally the diagnosis is confirmed by sonography and micturating cystourethrography.

Ditchfield, M. R., Grattan-Smith, J. D., de Campo, J. F., and Hutson, J. M. (1995). Voiding cystourethrography in boys: does the presence of the catheter obscure the diagnosis of posterior urethral valves? *Am. J. Roentgenol.*, **164**, 1233–5.

Reha, W. C. and Gibbons, M. D. (1989). Neonatal ascites and urethral valves. *Urology*, **33**, 468–71.

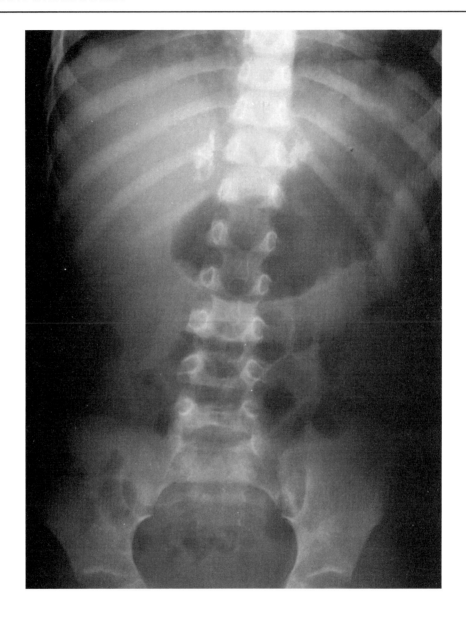

What coincidental abnormality is evident on the plain abdominal radiograph in this nine-year-old boy?

Adrenal calcification

There is bilateral paravertebral triangular-shaped calcification, at the level of T11 above the renal outlines, due to calcification in the adrenal glands.

Perinatal adrenal haemorrhage with subsequent calcification accounts for many cases of adrenal calcification on plain abdominal X-rays in children. There is no clinical consequence and adrenal function is normal. 'Idiopathic' calcification is occasionally discovered coincidentally when radiographs are performed for other reasons and the usual assumption is that unrecognized adrenal haemorrhage occurred at birth. Less commonly if a child recovers from meningococcal septicaemia with acute adrenal insufficiency (Waterhouse–Friderichsen syndrome) then calcification can ensue. In the developing world treated tuberculosis is a common cause of adrenal calcification.

A neuroblastoma typically causes a large mass lesion with unilateral rather than bilateral calcification in the suprarenal area. Wolman's disease is a rare cause of adrenal calcification and is usually fatal in the first year of life.

Ozmen, M. N., Aygun, N., Kilic, I. *et al.* (1992). Wolman's disease: ultrasonographic and CT findings. *Pediatr. Radiol.*, **22**, 541–2.

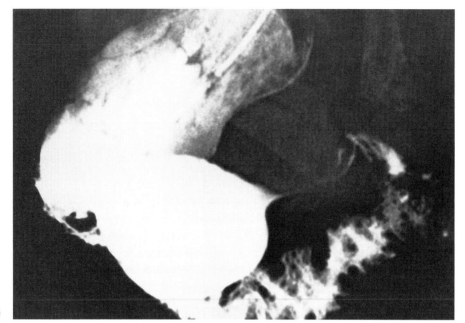

(a)

What abnormality on the barium meal examination accounts for this six-week-old boy's vomiting?

Hypertrophic pyloric stenosis

There is elongation (string sign) and narrowing of the pyloric canal due to the pyloric 'tumour'. A characteristic double track of barium connecting the antrum to the duodenal cap is evident. These findings were constant during the examination with associated delay in gastric emptying.

Hypertrophic pyloric stenosis (HPS) is a common cause of gastric outlet obstruction in infancy usually presenting at three to six weeks of age with non-bilious, projectile vomiting. The incidence is three times greater in boys than girls and full-term infants are more commonly affected than those born pre-term. The diagnosis is usually made clinically following a test feed when an olive-shaped pyloric mass is palpable to the right of the epigastrium. Gastric hyperperistalsis passing from left to right can be visible in the upper abdomen.

In doubtful cases, sonography is the investigation of choice (Fig. 3.9b). The pyloric area should be viewed continuously to ascertain whether the pyloric muscle hypertrophy is constant and the pyloric canal does not open properly. A pyloric muscle which is greater than 17 mm in longitudinal section, or greater than 4 mm in transverse section, is diagnostic of HPS. However, the ultrasound examination is a dynamic study and the diagnosis rests more on identifying pyloric muscle enlargement and lack of proper drainage through the pylorus than on actual measurements. In equivocal ultrasound cases or where paediatric ultrasound expertise is lacking, a barium meal study can be an alternative method of diagnosis typically showing shouldering at the antrum, constant elongation and narrowing of the pyloric canal.

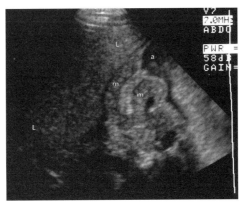

(b)

Longitudinal ultrasound of hypertrophic pyloric stenosis. Normal echogenic mucosa is seen between the thickened muscle. (a: antrum; m: pyloric muscle; L: liver).

Hernanz-Schulman, M., Sells, L. L., Ambrosino, M. M. *et al.* (1994). Hypertrophic pyloric stenosis in the infant without a palpable olive: accuracy of sonographic diagnosis. *Radiology*, **193**, 771–6.

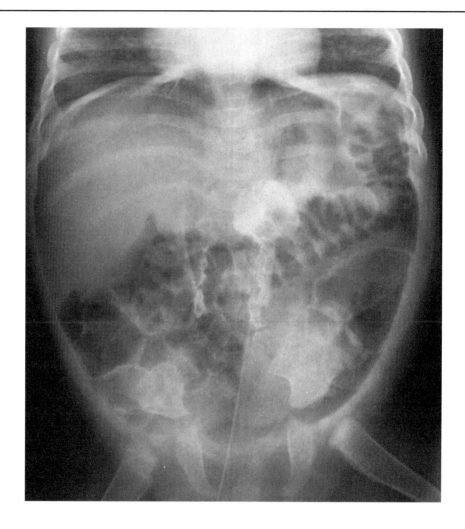

This infant has had a gastrostomy inserted. What complication has occurred?

Pneumoperitoneum

There are dilated gas-filled bowel loops in the lower abdomen with gas on both sides of the bowel wall (Rigler's sign) indicating free air in the peritoneal cavity. The pneumoperitoneum is also responsible for the large gas shadow in the upper abdomen with gas inferior to the diaphragm and free gas outlining both sides of the falciform ligament (curvilinear shadowing to the right of the upper lumbar spine). Spinal dysraphism is also present in the mid-lumbar region.

A relatively large amount of free air in the peritoneal cavity is necessary for visualization of a pneumoperitoneum on a supine abdominal radiograph. The main features on a supine film are air on both sides of the bowel wall, an abnormal collection of subhepatic gas, or a visible falciform ligament. Occasionally the lateral umbilical ligaments or umbilical arteries appear as an inverted V. When there is strong suspicion clinically, and the supine radiograph does not definitely confirm a perforation, then a decubitus film is recommended—smaller collections of free air can be confirmed with the patient in the left lateral decubitus position (with the right side up) when free air is seen separating the liver and abdominal wall.

Bray, F. J. (1984). The 'inverted V' sign of pneumoperitoneum. *Radiology*, **151**, 45–6.

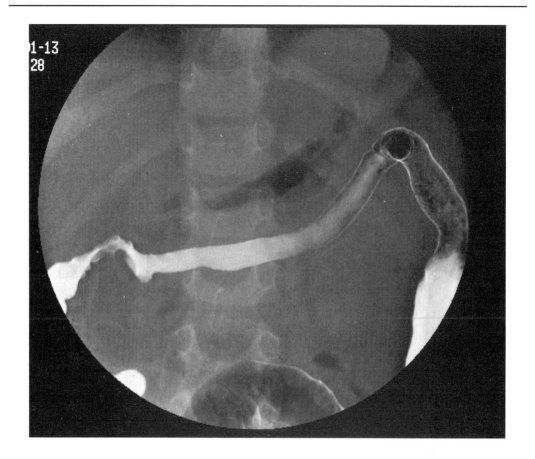

This four-year-old boy with cystic fibrosis had recurrent abdominal distension and pain. What lesion is evident on the barium enema?

Fibrosing colonopathy in cystic fibrosis

The transverse colon and splenic flexure region are narrowed and featureless with loss of the normal haustral pattern. In addition, there is narrowing with stricture formation at the hepatic flexure. At surgery severe narrowing with shrinkage of the ascending colon was also evident.

The distal intestinal obstruction syndrome or meconium ileus equivalent is the most common cause of recurrent colicky abdominal pain in children with cystic fibrosis (CF). This occurs secondary to impaction from viscid intestinal contents and faeces with partial bowel obstruction. In recent years submucosal and muscular fibrotic lesions of the colon have been reported in children with CF. This so-called 'fibrosing colonopathy' (there is no inflammation) is thought to be due to a toxic effect of a component of high strength replacement pancreatic enzymes, which have been discontinued as a result.

A standard barium enema will always show involvement and narrowing of the right side of the colon as the characteristic colonic fibrosis in this condition initially involves the caecal region with subsequent narrowing distally in the colon. Ultrasound, to identify patients with bowel wall thickening, has not been proved as a screening method and whenever this condition is suspected an enema is indicated.

Smyth, R. L., Ashby, D., O'Hea, U. *et al.* (1995). Fibrosing colonopathy in cystic fibrosis: results of a case control study. *Lancet*, **346**, 1247–51.

McHugh, K., Thomson, A., and Tam, P. (1994). Colonic stricture and fibrosis associated with high-strength pancreatic enzymes in a child with cystic fibrosis. *Br. J. Radiol.*, **67**, 900–1 (reprinted with permission).

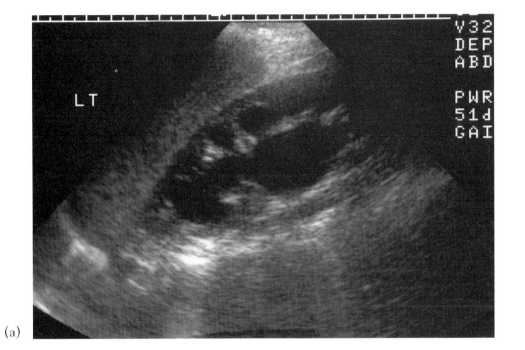

(a)

What abnormality is present on the longitudinal sonogram of the left kidney?

Hydronephrosis

Anechoic fluid distending the renal pelvis and calices is typical of hydronephrosis. Compare these findings with a normal right kidney (Fig. 3.12(b)).

The two major causes of hydronephrosis in childhood are vesicoureteric reflux and urinary tract obstruction. The indications for imaging children with urinary tract dilatation are dependent on the clinical circumstances and age of the patient. Ultrasonography is the recommended first imaging modality in all paediatric urinary tract disorders but it cannot reliably distinguish reflux from obstruction.

In neonates, hydronephrosis is often first identified on routine antenatal scanning. The investigation of hydronephrosis which is picked up antenatally is problematic as many cases are transient and of no clinical significance. At least two postnatal ultrasounds are generally recommended in these babies. The first examination is performed in the immediate newborn period to identify severe cases which need urgent urological work-up and another scan is done at around six weeks of age to ascertain if the urinary tract dilatation is persistent. As a general principle, if there is obvious caliceal dilatation or the renal pelvis diameter is greater than 15 mm then further investigations are necessary i.e. a micturating cystourethrogram (MCUG) to identify reflux.

In young children, hydronephrosis is often first detected in the setting of urinary tract infection. As vesicoureteric reflux is the most likely cause for hydronephrosis in these circumstances, a MCUG is the next recommended imaging study. In older children and adolescents in whom vesicoureteric reflux is unlikely, a Tc99m-MAG 3 renogram will be necessary to determine whether hydronephrosis is due to a non-obstructed baggy renal pelvis or due to functional obstruction at the pelvi-ureteric junction.

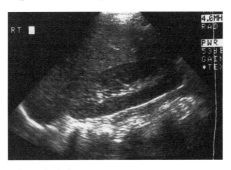

(b)

Normal longitudinal sonogram of the right kidney.

Hilton, S. W. and Kaplan, G. W. (1995). Imaging of common problems in paediatric urology. *Urol. Clin. North Am.*, **22**, 1–20.

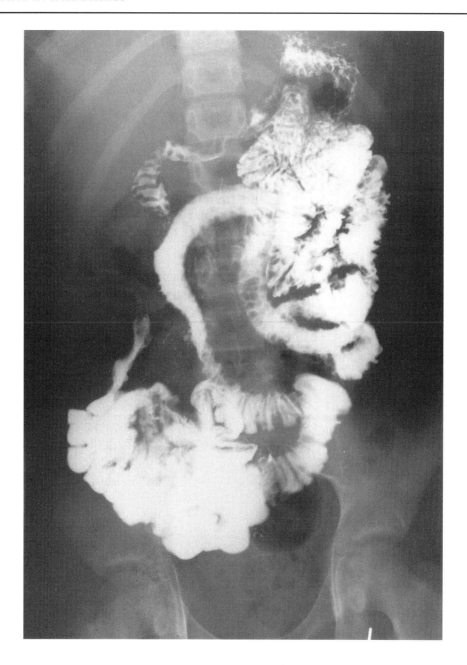

This child had recurrent cramping abdominal pain, growth retardation, and perianal fistulae. What diagnosis is confirmed on the barium follow-through study?

Crohn's disease

A small bowel loop in the central abdomen shows marked narrowing and mucosal thickening with wide separation from the other loops. Cobblestoning, narrowing, and ulceration is also present in some of the other small bowel loops on the left side of the abdomen.

Crohn's disease in childhood is uncommon with a prevalence of 1 in 10 000 but the incidence in this age group is believed to be rising. Diagnosis is often delayed, usually due to failure to consider the condition. Presentation is generally with a combination of abdominal pain, diarrhoea, weight loss, and growth retardation.

At least 70% of children with Crohn's disease have some small bowel involvement. A small bowel barium follow-through study is the investigation of choice with palpation and compression films (using a compression device) improving the accuracy of diagnosis. The terminal ileum is the most common site of involvement but children are much more likely than adults to have co-existent or isolated proximal small bowel disease. Skip lesions, which are short segmental lesions with normal bowel in between, are a characteristic finding in Crohn's disease of the small bowel. Oedema, mucosal thickening, and longitudinal fissures create a cobblestone appearance. A 'string sign' is a commonly used term on a barium study for a long segment of severely narrowed bowel. Stenoses and fistulae often complicate the course of the disease. Colonic Crohn's disease without small bowel involvement occurs in 10% of children.

Halligan, S., Nicholls, S., Bartram, C. I., and Walker-Smith, J. A. (1994). The distribution of small bowel Crohn's disease in children compared to adults. *Clin. Radiol.*, **49**, 314–16.

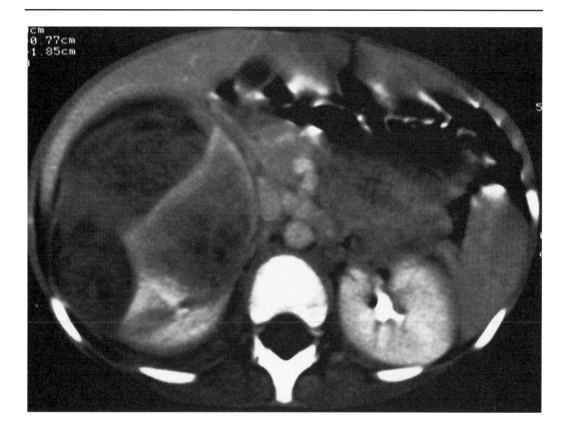

What lesion is present on the CT scan of a two year old with an abdominal mass?

Wilms' tumour

There is a well-encapsulated mass lesion arising from the right kidney with some normal enhancing renal tissue posterior to the tumour. The mass is of variable attenuation and lacks contrast enhancement. Note the normal enhancing left kidney with dense contrast in the left renal pelvis.

Wilms' tumour accounts for up to 12% of all childhood cancers and is the most common renal tumour in children. The most frequent presentation is with an abdominal mass. There is an increased incidence of Wilms' tumour in children with aniridia, cryptorchidism, and horse-shoe kidney. Hemihypertrophy, Beckwith–Wiedeman syndrome, and pseudohermaphroditism (Drash syndrome) also carry an increased risk.

Ultrasound is an excellent method for confirming the abdominal mass which can have an extremely variable echo pattern. The intrarenal origin of the lesion can usually be ascertained and ultrasound is particularly useful in assessing for extension of tumour thrombus into the inferior vena cava. CT can confirm these findings, particularly with large tumours when residual normal renal tissue can be difficult to identify. CT can also evaluate associated intra-abdominal lymphadenopathy and small foci of tumour in the opposite kidney, as approximately 5% of Wilms' tumours are bilateral at diagnosis. Differentiation of neuroblastoma from Wilms' tumour can be difficult with large tumours but the former tends to invade and encase the major abdominal vessels whereas Wilms' tumour typically displaces these structures without encasing the retroperitoneum. In Wilms' tumour the commonest site for metastases is the lungs with a 10% incidence of pulmonary metastases at presentation.

Reiman, T. A. H., Siegel, M. J., and Shackelford, G. D. (1986). Wilms' tumour in children: abdominal CT and US evaluation. *Radiology*, **160**, 501–5.

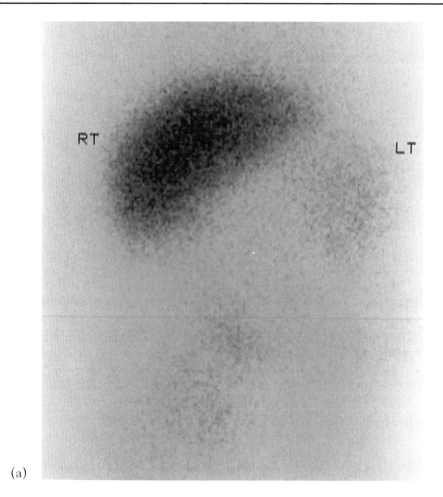

(a)

Static image from a Tc99m-HIDA scan taken eight hours post-injection. What abnormality is most likely in an infant with persistent cholestatic jaundice?

Biliary atresia

There has been uptake by the liver but no excretion of the radiopharmaceutical into the small intestine. Sequential images over a 24 hour period also confirmed a lack of excretion. A small amount of background activity in the kidneys and bladder is a normal finding. A normal Tc99m-HIDA study with excretion of the radiopharmaceutical into the gut is shown below for comparison (Fig (b)).

Biliary atresia and idiopathic neonatal hepatitis are overlapping conditions that probably represent two ends of a spectrum of obstructive cholangiopathies. They are clinically similar, often presenting with persistent jaundice and hepatomegaly in early infancy. Biliary atresia is now thought to be an acquired inflammatory disorder of the biliary tree. Jaundice usually begins in the first few weeks of life and increases gradually. Biliary atresia requires early surgery to prevent cirrhosis (portoenterostomy or liver transplantation) while neonatal hepatitis is treated medically.

Ultrasound cannot reliably differentiate between biliary atresia and neonatal hepatitis. The intrahepatic bile ducts are usually normal on ultrasound in both disorders but when dilated biliary atresia is more likely. Up to 10% of children with biliary atresia have associated anomalies such as polysplenia and an interrupted inferior vena cava.

In neonatal hepatitis there is often poor uptake of the injected isotope by the liver but excretion into bowel remains intact (pre-treatment with phenobarbital improves uptake and increases the accuracy of the examination). With biliary atresia on the other hand, uptake is excellent but excretion is lacking. Occasionally poor hepatocyte function can result in an inconclusive HIDA study and liver biopsy or cholangiography may be necessary to differentiate between the two disorders.

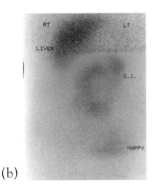

(b)   *Normal HIDA study. GI: gastrointestinal tract: nappy = diaper.*

Nadel, H. R. (1996). Hepatobiliary scintigraphy in children. *Semin. Nucl. Med.*, **26**, 25–42.

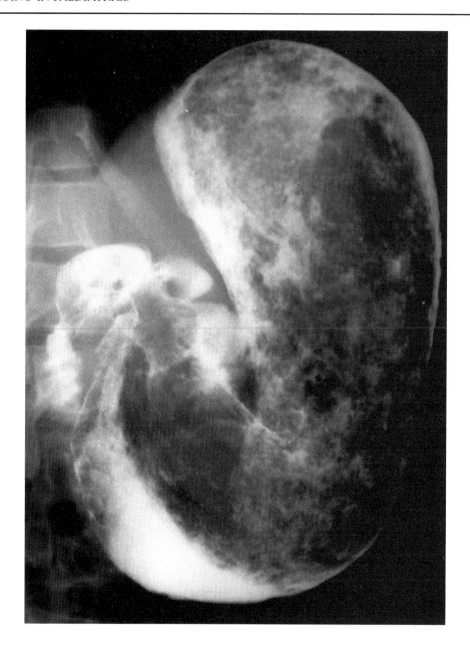

What abnormality is visible on the barium meal examination?

Bezoar (trichobezoar)

There is a large filling defect in the gastric lumen due to swallowed hair. The hair-ball (trichobezoar) has characteristic linear shadowing in the gastric antrum due to hair inter-mixed with adherent barium.

Ingested materials which accumulate in the stomach and form a non-opaque foreign body are termed bezoars. A trichobezoar or hair-ball is usually found in emotionally disturbed children and results from swallowed hair or fibres from a fur or wool garment. Weight loss, anaemia, halitosis, and anorexia are common accompanying features. Complications include upper gastrointestinal haemorrhage, gastric outlet, or small bowel obstruction. Lactobezoars, due to undigested milk curds, may also result in small bowel obstruction but are usually dissolved by fluid ingestion. However, surgical removal of trichobezoars is often necessary.

On plain radiographs, a gastric bezoar causes an intraluminal mass often with a mottled appearance due to air mixed within the foreign body. With barium ingestion the mass is outlined by barium adhering to the surface of the lesion. Gastric outlet obstruction or projection of the mass into the duodenum may be seen.

Newman, B. and Girdany, B. (1990). Gastric trichobezoars—sonographic and computed tomographic appearance. *Pediatr. Radiol.*, **20**, 526–7.

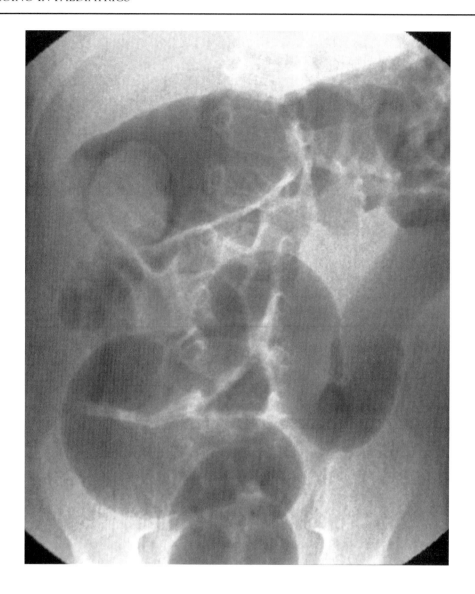

What procedure is being performed?

Pneumatic reduction of intussusception

An inflated Foley balloon is faintly visible in the rectum. Air has been inflated retrogradely and outlines the sigmoid, descending, and transverse colon. An intussusception is responsible for the mass lesion at the hepatic flexure.

The technique of pneumatic reduction involves air initially being introduced by a hand pump in puffs to allow observation of the movement of the advancing air column and to confirm or exclude the diagnosis of an intussusception. When confirmed, the intussusception is pushed back if possible by continuing to hand pump or by then switching to a specially designed mechanical pump at a pressure of 80 mmHg. The maximum recommended pressure is 100 mmHg—higher pressures than this can significantly increase the risk of perforation. Ultrasound can be used to diagnose an intussusception and is particularly helpful in doubtful cases.

Pneumatic reduction of intussusception is being increasingly used in many paediatric centres. It is gradually replacing hydrostatic (barium) reduction although barium reduction, properly performed, remains an excellent technique for reducing intussusceptions. Pneumatic reduction is faster, less messy, cheaper than hydrostatic reduction and may be more efficient, with success rates of 90% reported. Air enemas may lead to more bowel perforations as the pressure generated tends to be higher than with hydrostatic reductions. Intussusceptions that have been symptomatic for longer than 48 hours become increasingly difficult to reduce with the passage of time but the only absolute contraindications to pneumatic reduction are peritoneal inflammation, perforation, and shock.

Stein, M., Alton, D. J., and Daneman, A. (1992). Pneumatic reduction of intussusception: 5 year experience. *Radiology*, **183**, 681–4.

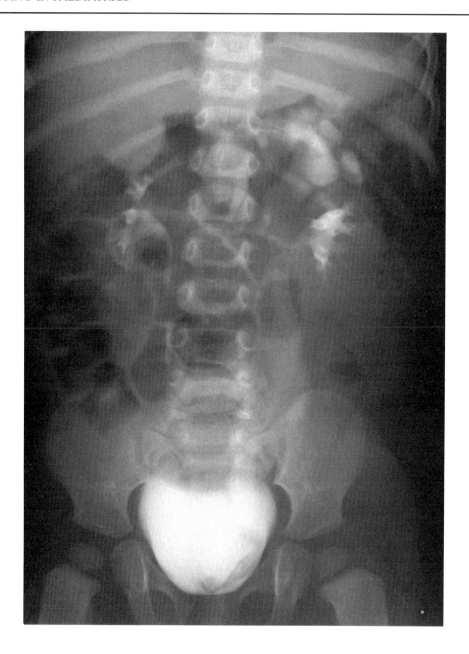

List the abnormalities on the intravenous urogram

1. *Duplex left kidney*
2. *Hydronephrotic upper moiety of left kidney*
3. *Hydroureter draining left upper moiety*
4. *Left ureterocele (causing filling defect on left of bladder)*

The majority of paediatric urinary tract disorders can now be comprehensively evaluated with a combination of ultrasound, nuclear medicine techniques, and micturating cystography. Consequently, the indications for an intravenous urogram (IVU) have diminished in recent years. However, the IVU still has a role to play in the assessment of abnormalities such as a duplex or horseshoe kidney, in the evaluation of enuresis due to a suspected ectopic ureter, and occasionally in the context of possible urinary tract calculi, papillary necrosis, or renal tuberculosis. No preparation is routinely necessary for an IVU and the use of purgatives in children should be avoided.

The IVU is superior to other techniques in defining the anatomical relationships of the two ureters draining a duplex system. The ureters may join or terminate separately. In a classic duplex collecting system, the ureter draining the upper moiety is ectopic and inserts below the orthotopic ureter. An ectopic ureter commonly inserts into the trigone, urethra, or vagina in females, or into the trigone or posterior urethra in males. Many ectopic ureters are complicated by a stenotic opening into the bladder or a ureterocele. Typically hydronephrosis of the upper moiety is due to obstruction at the ureterocele; hydronephrosis of the lower moiety is also common and is usually due to vesicoureteric reflux.

Young, D. W. and Lebowitz, R. L. (1986). Congenital abnormalities of the ureter. *Semin. Roentgenol.*, **21**, 172–87.

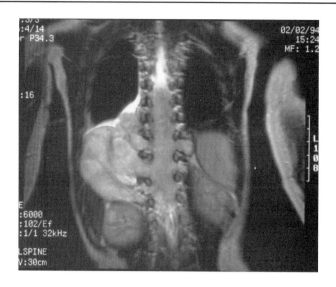

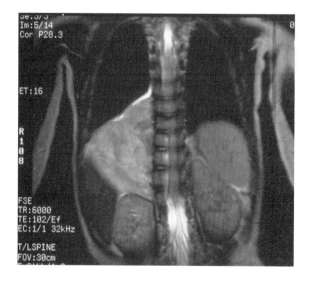

Coronal T2 weighted MRI sections through the chest and abdomen in a three year old with an abdominal mass. What is the diagnosis?

Neuroblastoma

There is a large mass lesion on the right side, superior to but separate from the right kidney which is displaced inferiorly. The mass has hyperintense T2 signal relative to the kidneys and spleen, and intraspinal extension of the tumour through widened intervertebral foramina is evident. Most of the spinal canal visible on the upper image is replaced by intraspinal tumour with a small amount of normal, bright T2 signal CSF seen superiorly. Extension of the tumour across the midline (stage 3 disease) is present with tumour extending to and through at least one left intervertebral foramen.

Neuroblastoma is the most common extracranial solid tumour in childhood. The disease affects young children with a peak incidence at two years of age. Neuroblastoma arises primarily in the abdomen in 60% of cases, most commonly in an adrenal gland. Intraspinal extension is uncommon with an adrenal primary but occurs in 15% of tumours arising in the sympathetic chain.

Ultrasound is the recommended first imaging modality for all children with a suspected abdominal mass. It can confirm the presence of a mass lesion and can guide further appropriate imaging. When feasible in small children, MRI is probably the single most useful imaging technique for the diagnosis and staging of neuroblastoma. Direct spread of tumour into the spinal canal and bone marrow metastases may also be identified. Skeletal metastases are routinely sought by Tc99m-MDP radionuclide bone scans. MIBG scans, usually labelled with Iodine-123, can also be used to detect metastatic disease or residual tumour following chemotherapy.

Ng, Y. Y. and Kingston, J. E. (1993). The role of radiology in the staging of neuroblastoma. *Clin. Radiol.*, **47**, 226–35.

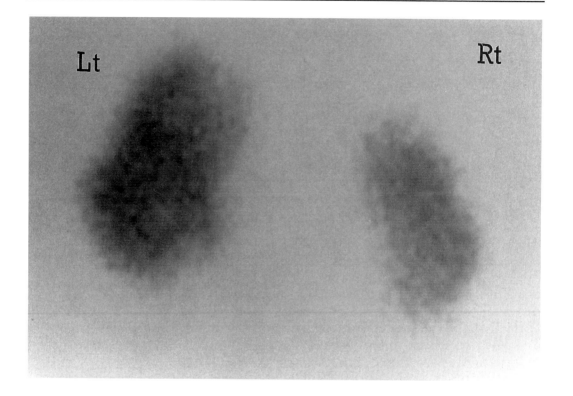

This child had a urinary tract infection (UTI) three months prior to this Tc99m-DMSA study. List two abnormalities.

1. *Scarring at the upper and lower poles of the left kidney*
2. *Atrophy of the right kidney (due to reflux nephropathy)*

The left kidney does not have a normal reniform outline due to scarring at the upper and lower poles. Chronic pyelonephritic damage has resulted in a shrunken right kidney. The right kidney contributes only 30% to overall renal function.

Tc99m-labelled DMSA (2,3 dimercaptosuccinic acid) has an affinity for the proximal convoluted tubules and accumulates in the renal cortex. This radiopharmaceutical is used solely for renal cortical imaging as very little renal excretion occurs. Static posterior and oblique images are routinely taken two hours after injection of the isotope.

DMSA scanning provides useful information regarding differential renal function and can be used to confirm reduced or non-function in a damaged or dysplastic kidney. In children, however, the major indication for DMSA imaging is in the investigation of UTIs. DMSA scans are performed most frequently in children up to 5 years of age approximately three months after a documented UTI—in the absence of interval infections, areas of diminished uptake indicate renal scarring. In the context of an acute UTI an area of diminished uptake could be due to acute pyelonephritis or a preceding renal scar. In chronic reflux nephropathy a small kidney with a deformed outline may be seen. There is an increasing trend towards performing DMSA studies during an acute UTI as it is the most sensitive method in establishing renal involvement (pyelonephritis) in this setting but a normal scan, however, does not exclude pyelonephritis.

Seigle, R. and Nash, M. (1995). Is there a role for renal scintigraphy in the routine initial evaluation of a child with a urinary infection? *Pediatr. Radiol.*, **25**, S52–3.

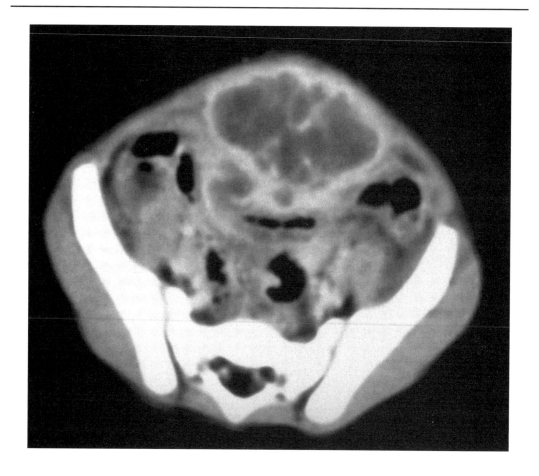

What abnormality is evident on the abdominal CT scan, after intravenous enhancement, in this one year old with fever and an abdominal mass?

Abscess: infected urachal cyst

The CT image shows a lower abdominal, anterior midline mass lesion with low attenuation fluid centrally (pus) and enhancing margins typical of an abscess collection.

Omphalovesical midline (urachal) anomalies are unusual congenital malformations and have been classified into four groups: a patent urachus, connecting the bladder to the umbilicus; urachal diverticulum (opening into the bladder); urachal sinus (opening at the umbilicus), and urachal cysts. The urachus is a remnant of the fibrosed allantoic stalk connecting the bladder and umbilicus, lying in the space of Retzius between the fascia transversalis and the peritoneum. A urachal sinus can present as a cord-like structure in the midline of the lower abdomen while the cystic lesions present as a mass which can occasionally become secondarily infected.

An appendiceal abscess or a cystic neoplasm could have an identical appearance to the abnormality on the CT scan in the illustration but the young age of the patient and the anterior midline location of the mass are more characteristic of an infected urachal cyst abscess.

Avni, E. F., Diard, D., and Schulman, C. C. (1988). Midline omphalo-vesical anomalies in children. Contribution of US imaging. *Urol. Radiol.*, **10**, 189–94.

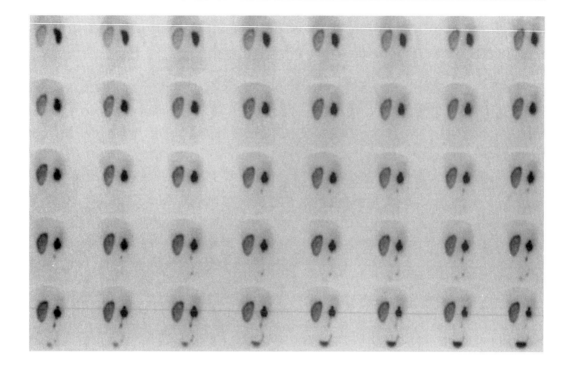

These 40 images are from consecutive 30 second frames from a dynamic Tc99m-MAG 3 renogram in a child with hydronephrosis. What abnormality is present?

Left pelvi-ureteric junction (PUJ) obstruction

There is normal uptake and excretion of the radiopharmaceutical by the right kidney (these are posterior images as is the convention in many nuclear medicine examinations). Delayed accumulation and washout from the larger, hydronephrotic left kidney is evident. In the bottom row of images the radiopharmaceutical can be seen delineating the right renal pelvis, right ureter, and bladder but no tracer is as yet visible in the left renal pelvis indicating delayed excretion on the left side.

Although ultrasound can easily diagnose hydronephrosis, it cannot reliably distinguish renal pelvic dilatation due to vesicoureteric reflux from a so-called PUJ obstruction. With a suspected functional PUJ obstruction a dynamic renogram with analogue images and time-activity curves are necessary. MAG 3 is preferred as the renographic agent in many centres as it is excreted by tubular secretion and has a higher extraction efficiency than Tc99m-DTPA, an alternative renographic agent. Frusemide, to effect a diuresis in dilated but not obstructed systems, is routinely administered in the evaluation of the dilated urinary tract. There is an increasing trend among paediatric surgeons to adopt a conservative approach in the management of functional PUJ obstruction in children, relying on serial renographic examinations with particular emphasis on divided function. Deteriorating function or function less than 30% (40% in some centres) in the hydronephrotic kidney are generally considered indications for pyeloplasty.

MAG 3, administered intravenously, is also used in co-operative, toilet-trained children as a method of indirect cystography, replacing conventional micturating cystography without the need for urethral catheterization. After the washout phase from the kidneys, the child voids in front of the gamma camera.

Eshima, D. and Taylor, A. (1992). Technetium-99m mercaptoacetyltriglycine: update on the new technetium-99m renal tubular function agent. *Semin. Nucl. Med.*, **22**, 61–73.

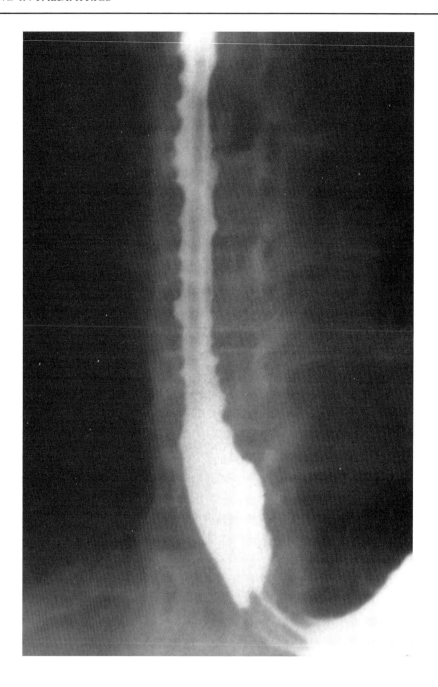

This child with dysphagia had recently swallowed an unidentified household fluid. What is the diagnosis?

Caustic oesophagitis

There is diffuse narrowing of the oesophagus with marked mucosal irregularity and ulceration. Diminished peristalsis was evident during the oesophagogram. A nasogastric tube traverses the oesophagus.

Ingestion of household cleaning products is nearly always accidental. Many cleaning substances are alkaline and corrosive and can produce a penetrating burn that may involve all layers of the oesophagus. In the acute phase, oesophageal perforation with mediastinitis can result. Mediastinitis may be suspected from chest radiographs by mediastinal widening, pneumomediastinum, or a pleural effusion.

Inspection of the mouth may show burns but their absence does not exclude an oesophageal lesion which should be sought with a contrast swallow examination. In the acute setting when the risk of perforation is high a standard non-ionic contrast medium rather than barium is recommended. Similarly, endoscopy is probably best avoided because of the perforation risk. Strictures of the oesophagus occur in up to 30% of cases as a late complication. A stricture may occur at any level of the oesophagus and can involve all or part of the circumference and a variable length. A stenotic rigid tube with abnormal peristalsis can result. Oesophageal shortening with contraction of scar tissue may lead to the development of a hiatus hernia with an increased risk of gastro-oesophageal reflux and pulmonary aspiration.

Nuutinen, M., Uhari, M., Karvali, T., and Kouvalainen, K. (1994). Consequences of caustic ingestion in children. *Acta. Paediatr.*, **83**, 1200–5.

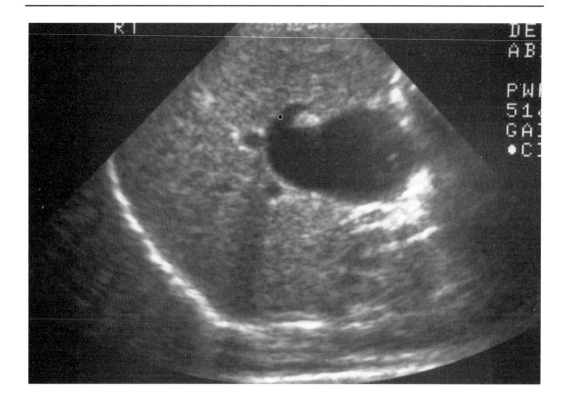

This infant had intermittent jaundice. What lesion is evident on the longitudinal sonogram of the liver?

Choledochal cyst

The anechoic (black) structure entering the inferior aspect of the liver represents fusiform dilatation of the common bile duct i.e. a choledochal cyst. The dilated common bile duct (CBD) is seen to merge with the left hepatic duct.

A choledochal cyst is characterized by cystic dilatation of the CBD and the majority of cases present within the first 10 years of life. Approximately one third of choledochal cysts present in infancy with larger lesions occasionally being detected on antenatal ultrasound. Presentation is highly variable and the symptoms are often intermittent. The classic triad of abdominal pain, jaundice, and a palpable mass is seen in 25% of patients; fever and ascending cholangitis are also frequent complications.

On sonography, a choledochal cyst appears as a well-defined, fluid-filled mass in the porta hepatis in continuity with the biliary tree but separate from the gall bladder. There are two major sub-types described: a type 1 cyst, which is the most common form, consists of fusiform dilatation of the CBD. A type 2 choledochal cyst is an eccentric diverticulum of the CBD. Secondary dilatation of the intra-hepatic bile ducts is found in about half of the affected patients. In addition to its role in diagnosis, ultrasound can also be useful in assessing the long-term complications of biliary stasis such as biliary cirrhosis and portal hypertension. Recurrent pancreatitis due to anomalous insertion of the CBD into the pancreatic duct is a recognized association.

Kim, O. H., Chung, H. J., and Choi, B. G. (1995). Imaging of the choledochal cyst. *Radiographics*, **15**, 69–88.

4. Musculoskeletal

Perthe's disease
Torus fracture and Salter–Harris classification
Ewing's sarcoma
Osteomyelitis
Langerhans cell histiocytosis of the skull
Congenital hip dislocation
Non-accidental injury with rib fractures
Discitis
Rickets
Slipped femoral capital epiphysis
Osteosarcoma
Mucopolysaccharidosis
Hip effusion
Lead poisoning
Osteochondroma
Fibrous dysplasia
Langerhans cell histiocytosis in a cervical vertebra
Osteogenesis imperfecta
Spondylolisthesis
Leukaemia

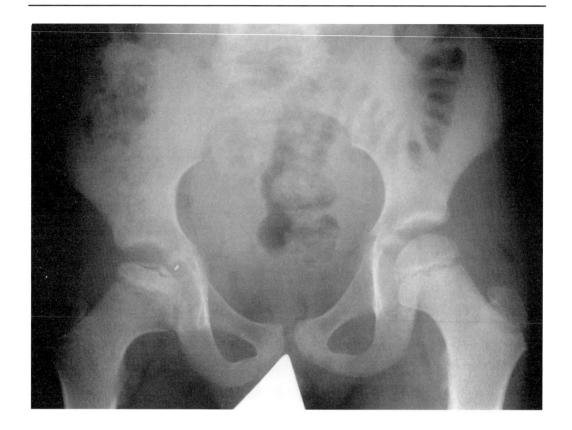

What abnormality is causing this child's limp?

Perthe's disease

There is widening of the joint space of the right hip with a subchondral lucency in the right femoral capital epiphysis. Sclerosis and partial collapse of the right femoral head are also visible. The left hip is normal.

Perthe's disease occurs between the ages of four and ten years, with a peak incidence at six years of age. Boys are affected four times as frequently as girls. Bilateral involvement occurs in 10% of cases with usually asymmetric disease in each hip. Common presenting complaints are pain in the groin or knee, often accompanied by a limp. Children with less than half the femoral head involved have a good prognosis, and those with greater than half the epiphysis affected tend to have more residual deformity. The goals of treatment are to maintain full range of movement at the hip joint with the femoral head contained within the acetabulum to minimize deformity.

The earliest plain radiographic feature of Perthe's disease is widening of the joint space of the hip, often best demonstrated on a frog-lateral view (abduction with external rotation). The frog-lateral film affords the best definition of the antero-lateral aspect of the proximal femoral epiphysis, where the changes of Perthe's disease usually originate. Subcortical lucency or fissuring in the epiphysis is another early radiographic sign which can progress to flattening, fragmentation, and sclerosis of the femoral head. Metaphyseal lucencies and broadening of the femoral neck are generally late features.

Bone scintigraphy with Tc99m-MDP is more sensitive than plain radiography in the detection of early cases when the avascular area is visible as a photopenic defect i.e. diminished uptake on the affected side. MRI is also superior to plain radiography early in the disease, but it is expensive and is usually reserved for problem cases.

Kaniklides, C., Lonnerholm, T., Morberg, A., and Sahlstedt, B. (1995). Legg–Calve–Perthe's disease. Comparison of conventional radiography, MRI, bone scintigraphy and arthrography. *Acta Radiol.*, **36**, 434–9.

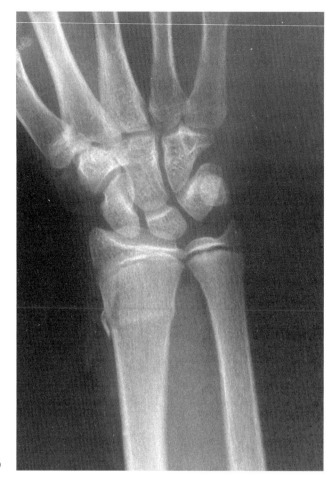

(a)

Name three fracture types in the distal left radius of this 12 year old who fell on to his outstretched hand.

1. Buckle (torus) fracture
2. Greenstick fracture
3. Salter–Harris type II epiphyseal fracture

Cortical buckling medially in the distal radius in association with a faint sclerotic band is due to a compression fracture. The break in the lateral cortex constitutes a greenstick lesion. A lucent fracture line extends from the lateral aspect of the compression fracture to the epiphyseal plate. Although no epiphyseal plate widening is evident on the AP radiograph, involvement of the epiphyseal plate should be assumed, and was confirmed on a lateral radiograph.

The inherent elasticity of the paediatric skeleton results in a propensity towards developing bowing and incomplete linear fractures. Compression failure on the concave side of a bending bone causes a buckle or torus fracture. A greenstick injury which is less common than, but can occur in association with, a torus fracture, is an incomplete fracture occurring on the convex side of a bone angulated beyond its limits.

The region of the epiphysis, epiphyseal plate, and metaphysis is involved in up to 15% of fractures of the long bones in children. As the epiphyseal plate is weaker than the surrounding ligaments and tendons, a variety of fractures through the epiphyseal plate region are recognized and classified (see Fig. b). Subsequent premature epiphyseal fusion can lead to angulation deformities or limb shortening.

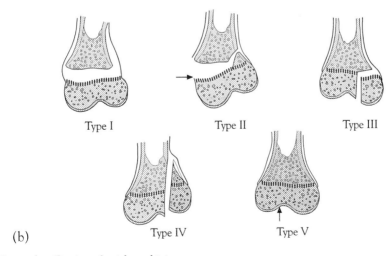

(b)

Salter–Harris classification of epiphyseal injury.

Rogers, L. F. and Poznanski, A. K. (1994). Imaging of epiphyseal injuries. *Radiology*, **191**, 297–308.

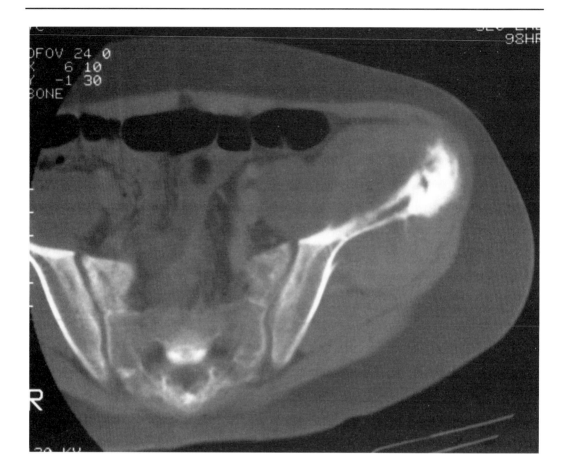

What lesion is visible on CT in the left iliac wing in this child with a palpable mass?

Ewing's sarcoma

There is a large soft tissue mass anterior and posterior to the left iliac wing. Loss of definition of the anterior cortex of the left iliac wing is evident with faint spiculated periosteal reaction and dense sclerosis in the lateral aspect of the iliac bone.

Ewing's sarcoma is one of the histological group of 'small round cell tumours' of childhood; the others include neuroblastoma, rhabdomyosarcoma, and lymphoma. Ewing's sarcoma can be osseous or soft tissue in origin and generally has a poor prognosis. Local pain, fever, and a soft tissue mass are common presenting complaints. It is frequently located in the pelvis, scapula, or ribs in older children and in the diaphysis of limb bones in early childhood.

Plain radiographs of the abnormality are initially necessary to characterize the lesion, to offer a probable diagnosis and to direct further imaging. On plain radiographs bone destruction with a moth-eaten or permeative pattern and a large adjacent soft tissue mass are frequent. Periosteal new bone formation in a classic 'onion-peel' or spiculated pattern is common in the long limb bones, but the periosteal reaction may have a variable appearance occasionally mimicking osteosarcoma or osteomyelitis. As a result, biopsy is necessary for histological confirmation.

MRI is recommended to assess the extent of marrow invasion, involvement of an adjacent epiphysis, and for assessment of the extra-osseous soft tissue component. MRI is also particularly useful during follow-up in assessing tumour response to chemotherapy, and in evaluating the possibility of limb salvage surgery. Radionuclide Tc99m-MDP bone scanning is used at initial presentation to identify or exclude distant skeletal metastases. Chest CT is also indicated for staging purposes as the lungs are the other common site for metastatic involvement at diagnosis.

Kauffman, W. M., Fletcher, B. D., Hanna, S. L., and Meyer, W. H. (1994). MR imaging findings in recurrent primary osseous Ewing sarcoma. *Magn. Reson. Imaging*, **12**, 1147–53.

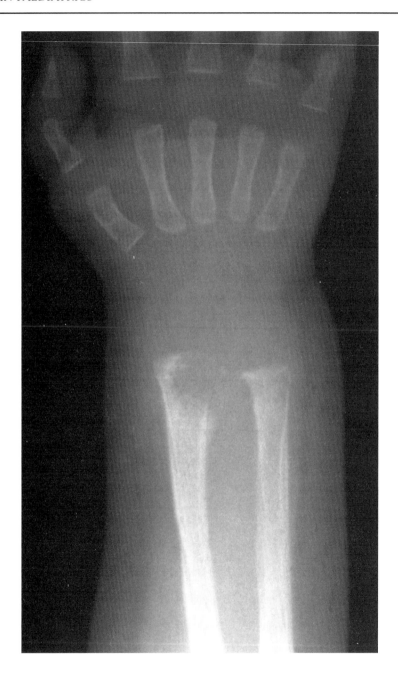

What is the diagnosis in this three week old with a swollen left wrist?

Osteomyelitis

The radiograph shows a well-defined lytic defect in the distal metaphysis of the left radius. The distal left forearm epiphyses and the carpal bones are cartilaginous and have not as yet ossified.

Acute osteomyelitis typically affects the metaphysis of long bones initially causing rarefaction, bone lysis, soft tissue swelling with later periosteal reaction and sclerosis. In the first year of life metaphyseal vessels pass through the growth plate into the cartilaginous epiphysis. Infants, therefore, are at particular risk of spread of infection from the metaphysis into the subarticular region and joint space. Metaphyseal infection can also lead to growth arrest and joint deformity, hence the need for prompt diagnosis. Inadvertent puncture of bone during venepuncture or arterial stabbing can occasionally lead to osteomyelitis particularly in infants. *Staphylococcus aureus* is the commonest causative organism in childhood osteomyelitis.

The radiographic changes of bone infection typically lag behind the clinical findings. A radionuclide bone scan (technetium 99m-MDP) will usually be positive prior to a demonstrable radiographic abnormality, and should be performed when there is strong clinical suspicion of osteomyelitis despite normal radiographs. A bone scan, which can image the entire skeleton can be particularly useful in the less common multifocal osteomyelitis which occurs in 22% of neonates and 7% of older children. MRI tends to be reserved for patients who have failed to respond to antibiotics and in whom surgery is contemplated, and in infections involving the epiphysis.

Jaramillo, D., Treves, S. T., Kasser, J. R. *et al.* (1995). Osteomyelitis and septic arthritis in children: appropriate use of imaging to guide treatment. *Am. J. Roentgenol.*, **165**, 399–403.

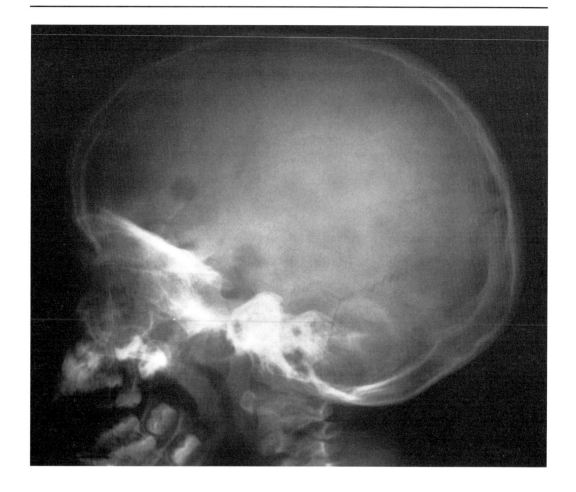

A lateral skull radiograph in a 3-year-old girl shows what abnormalities?

Lytic lesions due to Langerhans' cell histiocytosis

Two rounded lucencies in the skull vault with well-defined margins are visible–one in the frontoparietal region and the other in parietal bone superior to the lambdoid suture. The skull is otherwise normal.

Lytic skull vault lesions of variable size which have well-demarcated ('punched-out'), sometimes sclerotic, margins are typical of Langerhans' cell histiocytosis. Metastatic neuroblastoma and leukaemic involvement of the skull characteristically cause poorly defined lytic foci in the vault. The lesions of Langerhans' cell histiocytosis may be solitary or multiple and commonly affect the skull, spine, or long bones. Periosteal reaction in the shafts of long bones can occur if the cortex is eroded. A variety of systemic manifestations can occur in Langerhans' cell histiocytosis with diabetes insipidus and hypopituitarism being recognized complications of intracranial involvement.

Egeler, R. M. and D'Angio, J. (1995). Langerhans cell histiocytosis. *J. Pediatr.*, **127**, 1–12.

Jones, R. O. and Pillsbury, H. C. (1984). Histiocytosis X of the head and neck. *Laryngoscope*, **95**, 1031–5.

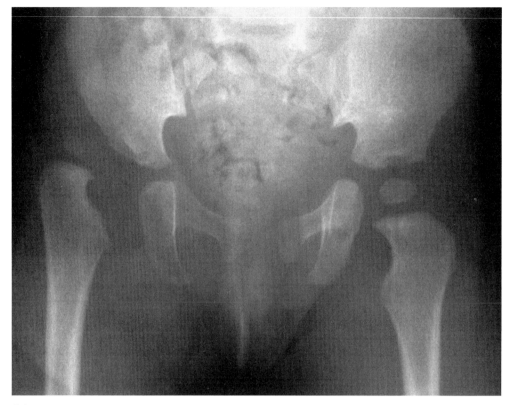

(a)

What abnormality is evident on the radiograph of the pelvis in this seven-month-old infant?

Congenital dislocation of the right hip

The right hip has dislocated superiorly forming a false acetabulum with the iliac bone above the true acetabulum. The slope of the right acetabulum is abnormal and the right femoral capital epiphysis is smaller than the left. The left hip is normal.

As many cases of congenital dislocation of the hip (CDH) may be acquired after birth, the term developmental dysplasia of the hip is an alternative description of this disorder. CDH has an incidence of between 2 and 8 per 1000 live births with a female:male ratio of approximately 6:1. It is more common after breech delivery and there is a familial tendency.

Ultrasound is the imaging modality of choice for assessing neonatal hip instability (Figs (b) and (c)). Two main approaches to hip ultrasound are used. A static method, pioneered by Graf, which produces a coronal image of the hip roughly equivalent to an AP radiograph is probably the more popular technique but it makes no attempt to assess stability. An alternative method is a dynamic study whereby the examiner attempts to dislocate the hip while scanning in the coronal and transverse planes. In essence, both methods satisfactorily evaluate acetabular morphology and the degree of coverage of the femoral head by the acetabulum.

The femoral capital epiphyses begin to ossify between three to six months of age. Plain radiographs become more reliable therefore in the assessment of CDH after six months, but are now mainly used in the evaluation of late presenting cases and in the follow-up of surgically treated patients. The position of the femoral head and the slope and development of the acetabulum are the critical findings on radiography. Although asymmetric femoral head ossification may be seen with unilateral CDH, it is an unreliable sign of instability.

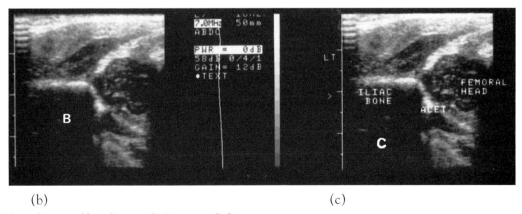

(b)   (c)

Normal neonatal hip ultrasound. Acet: acetabulum.

Harcke, H. T. (1995). The role of ultrasound in diagnosis and management of developmental dysplasia of the hip. *Pediatr. Radiol.*, **25**, 225–7.

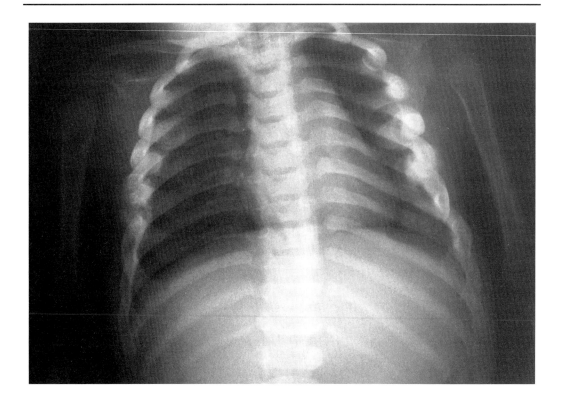

This five-month-old infant had an unexplained fracture through the mid-shaft of the right femur. The chest radiograph yielded other unexpected abnormalities. What lesions are evident and what is the likely diagnosis?

1. *Multiple healing rib fractures*
2. *Non-accidental injury*

Rib fractures with reparative callus formation are seen involving the left fourth to seventh ribs and the right third to sixth ribs on the anterior and lateral aspects. Faint periosteal new bone formation indicating injury is also evident along the lateral margin of the shaft of the left humerus.

Rib fractures in any location are rare accidental injuries in infants. Their occurrence generally requires severe trauma such as occurs in falls from a significant height or road traffic accidents. Birth injury and external cardiac massage rarely lead to rib fractures.

Fractures of the ribs are a relatively common finding in non-accidental injury, however. These fractures can occur anywhere along the rib arcs, and are difficult to identify in the acute phase. With reparative callus formation most rib fractures become visible within 10 to 14 days although fractures with markedly different amounts of callus formation suggest repeated injury. Fractures near the costovertebral articulation are relatively specific for non-accidental injury as they result from excessive anteroposterior thoracic compression and cannot occur from a direct blow.

Feldman, K. W. and Brewer, D. K. (1984). Child abuse, cardiopulmonary resuscitation and rib fractures. *Pediatrics*, **73**, 339–42.

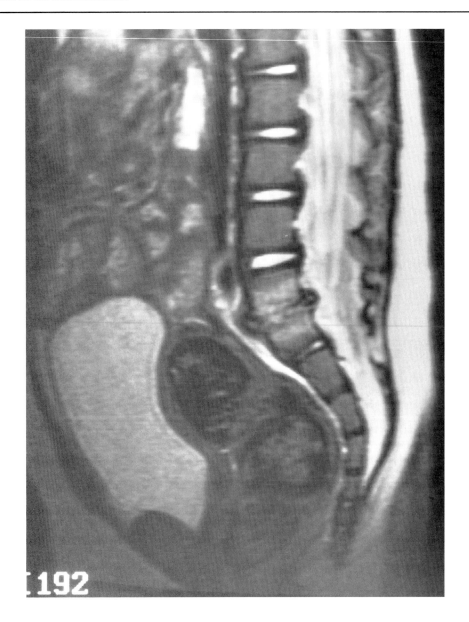

What is the diagnosis on the sagittal T2 weighted MR image of the lumbosacral spine in this four-year-old girl?

Discitis at L5/S1

There is loss of the normal signal of the L5/S1 disc (compare with the other intervertebral discs) with mild posterior L5/S1 disc protrusion. Increased T2 signal due to marrow oedema is visible in the two adjacent vertebral bodies.

Isolated discitis is not uncommon in childhood. From a practical viewpoint it can be regarded as part of a spectrum of infectious spondylitis ranging from discitis to vertebral osteomyelitis. Infection may originate in the disc or the vertebral end-plate with extension through the disc and subsequent involvement of the adjacent vertebral bodies. Infection is usually blood-borne and the common organisms responsible for vertebral osteomyelitis include *Staphylococcus aureus* and *Mycobacterium tuberculosis*. Discitis, however, can be an indolent condition particularly in younger children and a causative organism is often not identified either from blood cultures or a biopsy.

Plain radiographs typically show loss of disc space height with later loss of cortex from adjacent vertebral end-plates. An isotope bone scan can localize the site of abnormality in the spine, but is non-specific regarding aetiology as many different processes cause increased uptake of bone agent. An MRI examination is superior to other modalities in the evaluation of suspected discitis or vertebral osteomyelitis as it can easily assess inflammation in the disc and vertebral marrow, and can identify an epidural abscess which is a rare complication that may need drainage.

Szalay, E. A., Green, N. E., Heller, R. M. *et al.* (1987). Magnetic resonance imaging in the diagnosis of childhood discitis. *J. Pediatr. Orthop.*, **7**, 164–7.

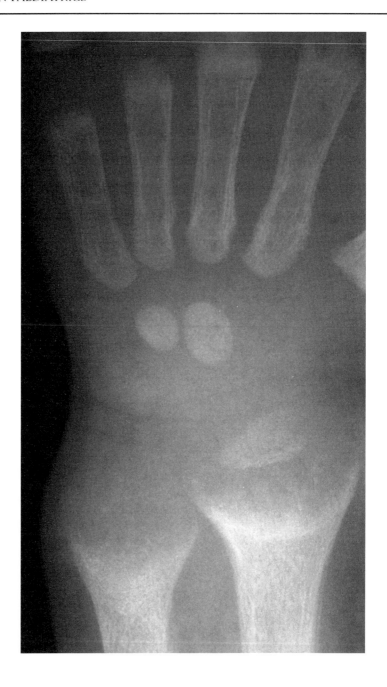

What metabolic bone disorder is responsible for the appearances at the left wrist?

Rickets

There is rarefaction, splaying, and cupping of the metaphyses of the distal radius and ulna.

Inadequate dietary intake of vitamin D and reduced sunlight exposure are common causes of rickets. Other causes include long-term anticonvulsant therapy, chronic renal and hepatic disorders, inherited vitamin D-dependent rickets, and X-linked hypophosphatemic vitamin D-resistant rickets. All types share common radiographic features.

Splaying, cupping, and irregularity of the metaphses are evident in virtually all cases of rickets. These changes are best appreciated at the growing ends of long bones such as the distal radius and ulna in infants who crawl, and around the knees in ambulant children. However, the whole skeleton can be affected with widespread coarsening of the trabecular pattern, osteopenia, and cortical thinning. Bowing of the lower limbs and fractures may occur. Splaying and cupping of the anterior ribs at the costochondral junctions leads to a rickety rosary which may be palpable clinically. The skull may become decalcified with frontal bossing.

The effects of therapy should be monitored by radiography at appropriate intervals. As the therapeutic doses of vitamin D are relatively high in vitamin D-resistant rickets, these children merit more frequent radiographic assessment including regular renal ultrasound examinations because of a risk of nephrocalcinosis with long term high dose vitamin D treatment.

Pitt, M. J. (1991). Rickets and osteomalacia are still around. *Radiol. Clin. North Am.*, **29**, 97–118.

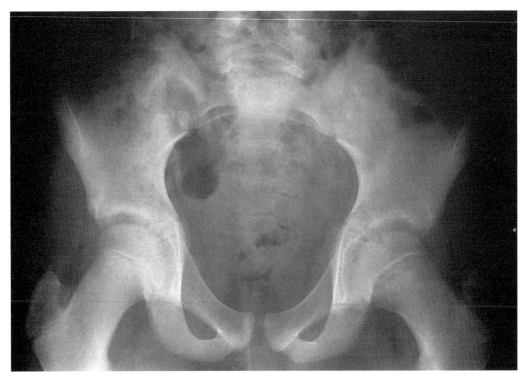

(a)

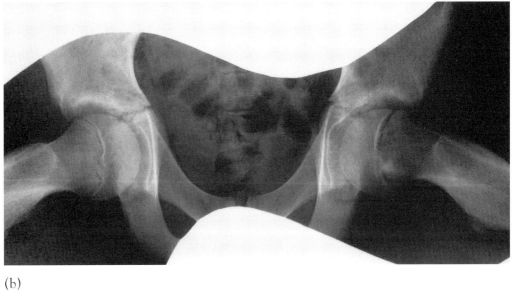

(b)

What abnormalities on the AP and frog-lateral films are causing this adolescent's hip pain?

Bilateral slipped femoral capital epiphyses

(a) There is a probable slip of the left capital femoral epiphysis on the AP radiograph but the right femoral head appears essentially normal. (b) The frog-lateral film demonstrates an inferior slip of the left capital femoral epiphysis with an early slip on the right side also i.e. bilateral involvement.

A slipped femoral capital epiphysis (SFCE) usually occurs around the onset of puberty. Consequently, the peak incidence is earlier in girls (11–12 years) than in boys (14 years). Nevertheless boys are affected more frequently with a male:female ratio of approximately 2:1. Bilateral involvement occurs in 20–40% of cases. Overweight adolescents are particularly susceptible. The onset is usually insidious, with pain in the hip or knee or a limp being frequent presenting complaints.

The initial signs of a slipped epiphysis can be quite subtle on an AP radiograph of the pelvis. Widening of the growth plate or greater than 2 mm difference in epiphyseal height when compared to the contralateral hip may be visible in unilateral cases. A straight line drawn along the lateral margin of the femoral neck should normally transect the superior aspect of the femoral epiphysis—loss of intersection by this lateral cortical line with the epiphysis suggests a slip. Similarly, the medial third of the upper femoral neck should overlie the posterior aspect of the acetabulum. A slipped epiphysis may also be suspected by displacement of the femoral neck away from the acetabulum.

The separation or displacement of the epiphysis on the metaphysis is virtually always in a posterior direction and is most easily appreciated on a frog-lateral radiograph (abduction with external rotation) which should be performed in all adolescents with hip pain. In 10% of cases no abnormality is detected on the AP film but the frog-lateral radiograph is invariably diagnostic with characteristic medial and inferior displacement of the epiphysis. Occasionally a slip occurs acutely after trauma when the injury is generally regarded as a transepiphyseal fracture (Salter–Harris type I p. 141).

Loder, R. T. (1995). Slipped capital femoral epiphysis in children. *Curr. Opin. Pediatr.*, **7**, 95–7.

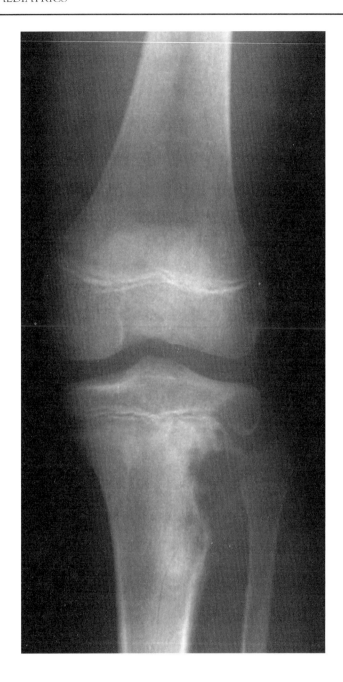

A painless lump was present over the left knee. What is the diagnosis?

Osteosarcoma

There is eccentric lytic destruction in the lateral aspect of the proximal metaphysis of the left tibia. There is ill-defined sclerosis in the metaphysis medial to the lesion with poor definition to the margins of the abnormality ('wide zone of transition') indicating an aggressive bone lesion. Lucency in the lateral aspect of the proximal tibial epiphysis was confirmed on MRI to be secondary to tumour extension across the epiphyseal plate.

The incidence of osteosarcoma is maximal in the second and third decades with a predilection for long bones, particularly around the knees. Osteosarcoma is characteristically located eccentrically in the metaphysis. Osteosclerosis with dense new bone formation and a variable pattern of periosteal reaction e.g. Codmans's triangle (spiculated periosteal new bone) is the classical radiographic appearance of osteosarcoma. In many tumours bone lysis predominates. Extension of tumour into the adjacent soft tissues causing a palpable lump is frequent. Chronic sclerosing osteomyelitis can be indistinguishable radiographically from a bone sarcoma, although the former usually lacks a soft tissue mass and characteristically has a 'tunnel' of bone destruction within it.

Despite the correct diagnosis of many bone tumours often being possible on radiographs alone, plain radiographs and other imaging modalities are imprecise with respect to exact histology and so a bone biopsy is essential in all cases. Additional MR imaging is recommended to delineate the exact extent of intramedullary spread of tumour, to assess tumour extension into the epiphysis and adjacent soft tissues, and to act as a baseline study in the evaluation of tumour response to chemotherapy. MR can occasionally identify skip lesions elsewhere in the marrow at presentation. Distant skeletal metastases are routinely sought at initial diagnosis by Tc99m-MDP radionuclide bone scanning. In addition, chest CT is also used routinely for staging the tumour at presentation, to identify pulmonary metastases which is metastatic osteosarcoma can occasionally calcify.

Kumar, R., Ruppert, D., Madewell, J. E., and Lindall, M. M. Jr. (1987). Radiographic spectrum of osteogenic sarcoma. *Am. J. Roentgenol.*, **148**, 767–72.

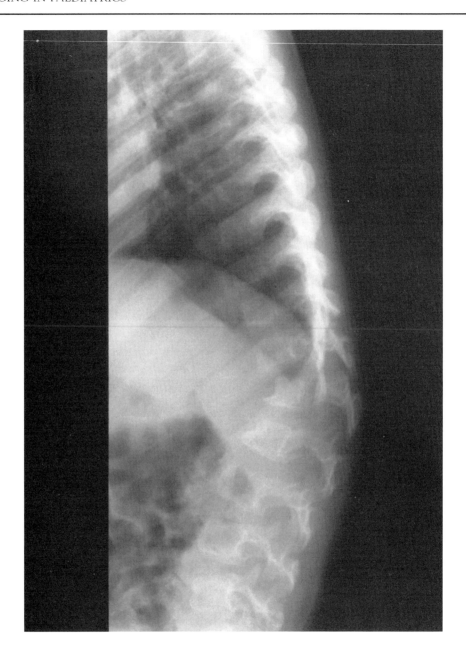

What storage disorder is responsible for the abnormality of vertebral body shape visible on the lateral thoraco-lumbar spine radiograph?

Mucopolysaccharidosis: Hurler's syndrome

There is anterior beaking of the lower aspects of the upper two lumbar vertebrae. In addition, there is posterior displacement of the first beaked vertebra (L1) relative to T12 with a thoraco-lumbar kyphosis.

The mucopolysaccharidoses are a heterogenous group of conditions resulting from complex disorders of carbohydrate metabolism. The descriptive term 'dysostosis multiplex' is given to the radiologic features seen in many children who have a mucopolysaccharidosis (MPS), except Morquio's syndrome which has specific radiologic findings. Hurler's syndrome (MPS 1-H) is an autosomal recessive disorder due to a deficiency of α-L-iduronidase. The patients are normal at birth but around the end of the first year there is a marked decrease in linear growth. Without treatment the condition is progressive with coarsening of the facial features (gargoylism), mental retardation, hepatosplenomegaly, and ultimately death from cardio-respiratory complications.

Hurler's syndrome shows many of the features of dysostosis multiplex and can be regarded as the prototype MPS from a radiographic viewpoint. These features include thickening of the skull vault with a large J-shaped sella, thickening of the ribs which taper posteriorly (oar-shaped), flaring of the pelvis with small iliac bones, short limb bones with broad metacarpals and metatarsals which have pointed proximal ends. Achondroplasia can also cause antero-inferior vertebral body beaking but in that condition there is invariably shortening of the pedicles in the neural arch with spinal canal narrowing.

Eggli, K. D. and Dorst, J. P. (1986). The mucopolysaccharidoses and related conditions. *Semin. Roentgenol.*, **21**, 275–94.

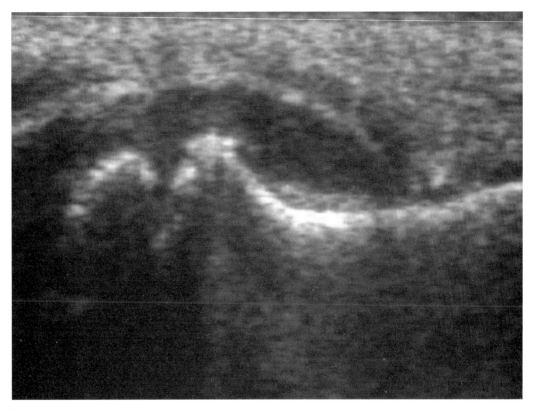

(a)

This is an ultrasound examination of the left hip of a four-year-old boy who presented with a limp. What is the diagnosis?

Hip joint effusion: secondary to transient synovitis

This sonogram is produced by placing a linear transducer longitudinally over the anterior hip with the child lying supine and the legs extended. The capsule of the hip joint normally has a concave contour paralleling the femoral neck (see diagram below). With an effusion the capsule bows anteriorly. An antero–posterior diameter between the femoral neck and the capsule greater than 5 mm or a 2–3 mm difference on either side is indicative of an effusion.

Transient synovitis causing an irritable hip usually presents in children between the ages of three and nine years. Limp or pain in the knee are common presenting symptoms.

Sonography is very sensitive in the detection of hip effusions. Anechoic collections i.e. those which lack internal echoes are generally serous, whilst purulent collections are often echogenic. A septic arthritis can be difficult to diagnose clinically – an ultrasound examination however cannot reliably differentiate a transient synovitis from a septic arthritis. Consequently, in some centres all hip joint effusions in children are aspirated under local anaesthesia with ultrasound guidance. Plain radiographs are inaccurate in the assessment of hip effusions (widening of the joint space is a late and unreliable sign) but can occasionally demonstrate an unsuspected adjacent osteomyelitis or Perthe's disease.

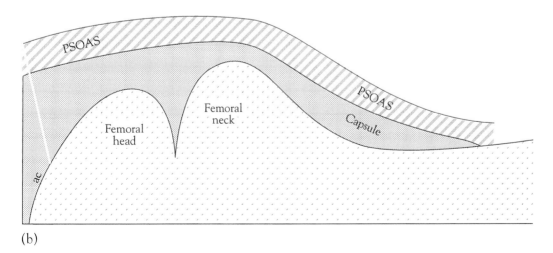

(b)

Diagram of normal longitudinal hip ultrasound. ac: articular cartilage.

Berman, L., Fink, A. M., Wilson, D., and McNally, E. (1995). Technical note: identifying and aspirating hip effusions. *Br. J. Radiol.*, **68**, 306–10.

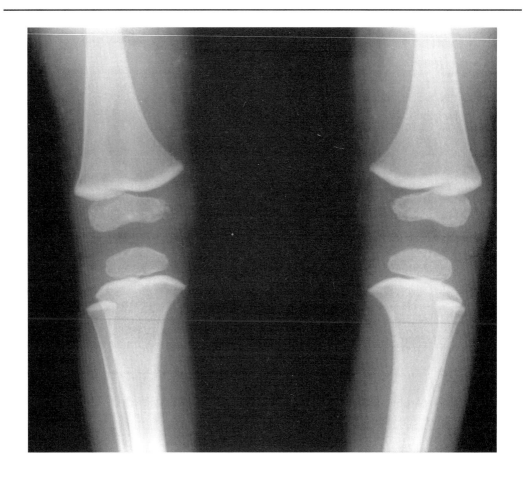

What is causing the changes at the knee joints?

Lead poisoning

Dense sclerosis is noted in the metaphyses adjacent to the growth plates of the distal femur, proximal tibia and fibula bilaterally. Although some metaphyseal sclerosis can be seen in the normal paediatric skeleton, sclerosis in the proximal fibula is abnormal.

Lead poisoning is found mainly in children who ingest lead-containing paint from old buildings or repainted furniture. The habit is a form of pica and is more common in deprived or neglected children.

Dense transverse metaphyseal lines develop following exposure to lead or other heavy metals. The transverse sclerotic bands can be seen throughout the growing skeleton particularly at the hands, ankles, and knees. An abdominal radiograph can confirm the diagnosis when radio-opaque flakes of paint are present within the intestine. Dense metaphyseal sclerosis is not, however, specific for heavy metal poisoning and it can be seen in other conditions including the healing phase of treated rickets or leukaemia.

Woolf, D. A., Riach, I. C., Derweesh, A., and Vyas, H. (1990). Lead lines in young infants with acute lead encephalopathy: a reliable diagnostic test. *J. Trop. Pediatr.*, **36**, 90–3.

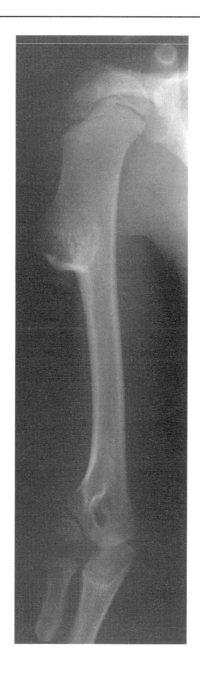

What is causing the lump on this child's upper right arm?

Osteochondroma

Expansion of the lateral aspect of the proximal right humerus is present with no evidence of osteolysis. The lesion is continuous with the medullary cavity, and the appearances are typical of a sessile osteochondroma.

Osteochondromas are cartilage-based benign tumours which project from the surface of a bone. They may be sessile or pedunculated; the latter are also called bony exostoses. An osteochondroma may present as a painless lump or be picked up incidentally on a radiograph performed for an unrelated reason. Occasionally they may impinge on blood vessels or nerves. Growth of these lesions ceases with skeletal maturation. There is an increased incidence of osteochondromas at the site of previous irradiation in patients who have had radiotherapy for childhood cancer.

Osteochondromas originate in the metaphysis near the epiphyseal plate and characteristically point away from the joint. These tumours have a cartilaginous cap which is not visible on plain radiographs, and the medullary cavity of the tumour is always in continuity with the parent bone. Sites of predilection include the proximal humerus, hip, and knee although lesions occasionally arise in flat bones. Diaphyseal aclasis, which can result in widespread bone modelling deformities, is an autosomal dominant condition characterized by multiple exostoses.

Shore, R. M., Poznanski, A. K., Anandappa, E. C., and Dias, L. S. (1994). Arterial and venous compromise by an osteochondroma. *Pediatr. Radiol.*, **24**, 39–40.

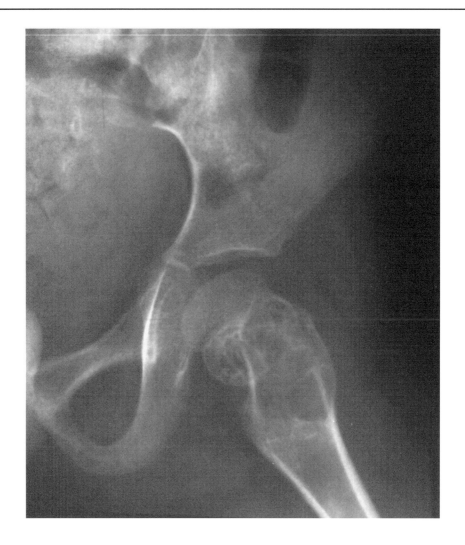

What lesion is evident in the proximal left femur?

Fibrous dysplasia

There is a lucent lesion deforming and causing mild expansion of the femoral neck and proximal metaphysis. The area of abnormality has a well-defined demarcation from normal bone (a narrow 'zone of transition') indicating a non-aggressive or benign bone process. The epiphysis is normal.

Fibrous dysplasia is a benign condition of unknown aetiology that can affect any part of the paediatric skeleton. There are essentially two types: monostotic (affecting only one bone) and polyostotic fibrous dysplasia. McCune–Albright syndrome, which occurs mainly in females, comprises polyostotic fibrous dysplasia in association with skin pigmentation and precocious sexual development.

In the long bones, lytic lesions predominate. These foci of fibrous dysplasia tend to have well-defined margins, often expand the bone and may have an internal ground-glass appearance. Modelling deformities and pathological fractures are common. With femoral neck involvement coxa vara and a so-called 'shepherd's crook' deformity are frequently seen. In the skull there is often thickening and sclerosis of the skull vault, base and facial bones with obliteration of the paranasal sinuses. The lesions of fibrous dysplasia characteristically show intense uptake of radiopharmaceutical on Tc99m-MDP bone scintigraphy such that assessment of suspected associated fractures should be with plain radiographs.

Lucas, E., Sundaram, M., and Boccini, T. (1995). Radiologic case study. Polyostotic fibrous dysplasia. *Orthopedics*, **18**, 311–13.

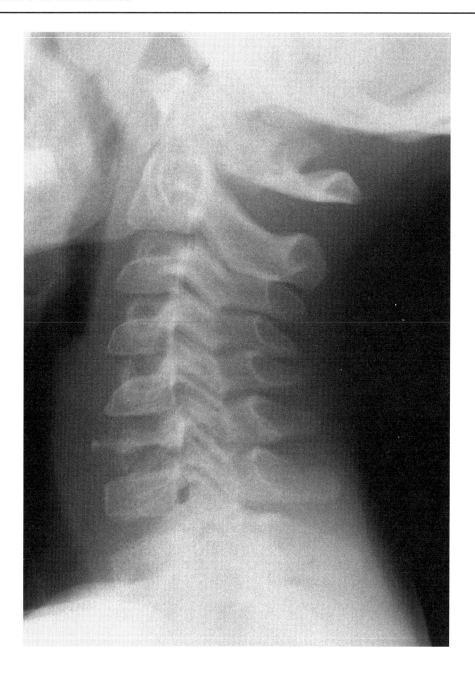

What abnormality is evident on the lateral cervical spine film in this five year old? What is the probable aetiology?

1. Vertebra plana
2. Langerhans' cell histiocytosis

There is complete flattening of the C6 vertebral body with an increase in the antero–posterior diameter. The adjacent disc spaces and end-plates of C5 and C7 are normal. There is no discernible prevertebral soft tissue swelling.

True vertebra plana is usually caused by infiltration of a vertebra by Langerhans' cells histiocytosis. Histiocytosis X, eosinophilic granuloma, Letterer–Siwe disease, and Hand–Schüller–Christian syndrome are related conditions now grouped under the term Langerhans' cell histiocytosis. A solitary skeletal lesion can affect any bone but involvement of a vertebral body with preservation of the neural arch is characteristic. Enroachment on the spinal canal is unusual.

Normal disc spaces and adjacent end-plates in the illustration essentially rule out infection as a cause of the vertebral collapse. Other causes of a collapsed vertebra, particularly leukaemia, should be excluded. The lesions of Langerhans' cell histiocytosis do not as a rule avidly take-up radionuclide bone agent, and so in the search for suspected multiple lesions a radiographic skeletal survey is preferred.

George, J. C., Buckwalter, K. A., Cohen, M. D., *et al.* (1994). Langerhans' cell histiocytosis of bone: MR imaging. *Pediatr. Radiol.*, **24**, 29–32.

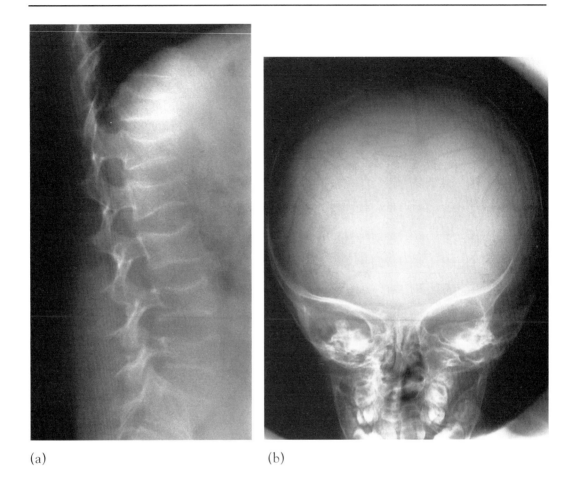

(a)   (b)

A lateral lumbar spine film and an anteroposterior skull radiograph in two children with the same disorder. What is the unifying diagnosis?

Osteogenesis imperfecta

The vertebrae are osteoporotic with multiple biconcave deformities indicating partial collapse of the vertebral bodies. The skull contains multiple wormian (intrasutural) bones.

Osteogenesis imperfecta is due to an abnormality of type I collagen and is characterized by osteoporosis, bone fragility, and fractures. Most cases result from autosomal dominant inheritance or new mutations. Spontaneous improvement is commonly observed in adolescence with a reduction in the frequency of fractures.

Osteogenesis imperfecta is usually classified into four types with additional subtypes depending on the presence or absence of dental abnormalities. Type 1 is the most common form (70%) with generally mild to moderate bone fragility. Fractures occur most frequently in pre-school age children but a few have fractures at birth. Osteoporosis with thinning of the bony cortex is usually evident. Blue sclera and wormian bones are characteristically also present. Type 2 is usually lethal *in utero* or in the neonatal period. Severe bone changes are seen in the type 3 disorder with fractures at birth and throughout childhood with bowing deformities and kyphoscoliosis. Type 4 is characterized by mild to moderate bone fragility with fractures at birth in up to 30%. Wormian bones are present but the sclera are usually normal.

Ablin, D. S., Greenspan, A., Reinhart, M., and Grix, A. (1990). Differentiation of child abuse from osteogennesis imperfecta. *Am. J. Roentgenol.*, **154**, 1035–46.

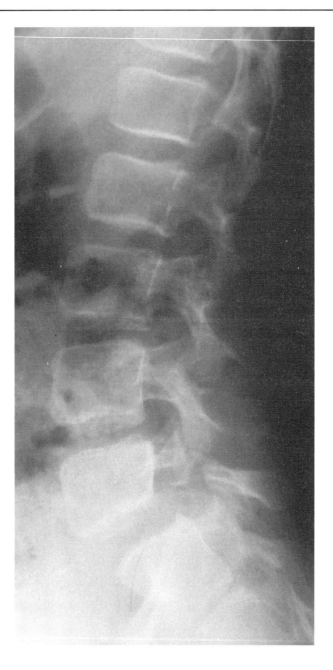

(a)

What is the cause of this child's back pain?

Spondylolisthesis at L5/S1

There is forward slip of L5 on S1 due to a defect in the pars interarticularis bilaterally at L5.

Spondylolisthesis is the forward slip of one lumbar vertebra on another. The pars interarticularis is the superior aspect of the inferior articular process immediately posterior to the pedicle of a lumbar vertebra (see diagram). A defect in the pars is called a spondylolysis. The majority of pars defects are considered stress fractures and are more frequently seen in young athletes usually at the L4/5 or L5/S1 level. Presentation is usually with vague low back pain.

Defects in the pars are difficult to detect in the early stages and are more easily identified on oblique projections. Bilateral pars defects are necessary for spondylolisthesis to take place which when severe can lead to an excessive lordosis. Anterior displacement of one vertebral body, usually the upper vertebra, on another is best appreciated on lateral radiographs. When a spondylolisthesis occurs, ventral slipping of the body, pedicles, and superior articular processes of the involved vertebra takes place while the spinous process, laminae, and inferior articular processes remain in position. The neural canal is widened and so neurological complications are uncommon.

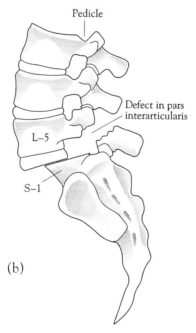

Pedicle

Defect in pars interarticularis

L-5

S-1

(b)

Spondylolisthesis at L5/S1.

Jinkins, J. R., Matthes, J. C., Sener, R. N., *et al.* (1992). Spondylolysis, spondylolisthesis and associated nerve root entrapment in the lumbosacral spine: MR evaluation. *Am. J. Roentgenol.*, **159**, 799–803.

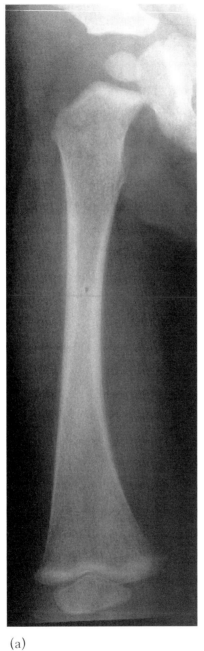
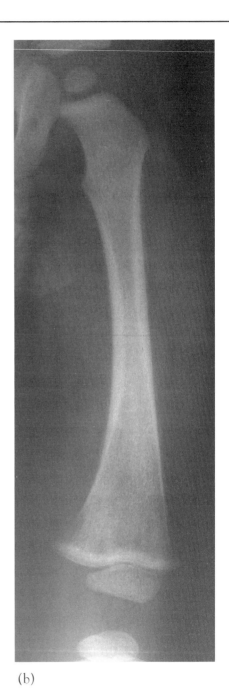

(a)   (b)

This child had bilateral lower limb pains. What blood disorder is responsible for the changes in both femora?

Leukaemia

There is faint periosteal reaction along the shafts of the femora due to leukaemic infiltration. In addition, both distal femoral metaphyses are abnormal with ill-defined areas of translucency (compare to the normal proximal metaphyses), also secondary to infiltration.

The classic skeletal manifestation of leukaemia on plain radiographs is transverse metaphyseal lucent bands adjacent to the growth plates in the long bones. These translucencies are not specific for leukaemia and may be seen in a number of other severe or chronic illnesses. Less commonly, vertebral collapse, focal osteolytic lesions, or generalized osteoporosis can be seen at presentation. Periosteal new bone formation with ill-defined areas of translucency in the metaphyses and skull are well recognized in leukaemia but metastatic neuroblastoma can produce similar radiographic findings. Due to earlier diagnosis and treatment bone changes are less commonly seen now in childhood leukaemia, and the skeletal changes generally resolve with successful therapy.

Benz, G., Brandeis, W. E., and Willich, E. (1976). Radiological aspects of leukaemia in childhood: an analysis of 89 children. *Pediatr. Radiol.*, **2**, 201–13.

5. Neuroradiology

Adrenoleucodystrophy
Acute extradural haematoma
Thalassaemia
Retinoblastoma
Agenesis of the corpus callosum
Cerebral infarct
Skull fracture
Medulloblastoma
Encephalitis
Craniopharyngioma
Hypoxic-ischaemic encephalopathy
Tuberous sclerosis
Vein of Galen malformation
Acute on chronic subdural haematoma
Craniosynostosis

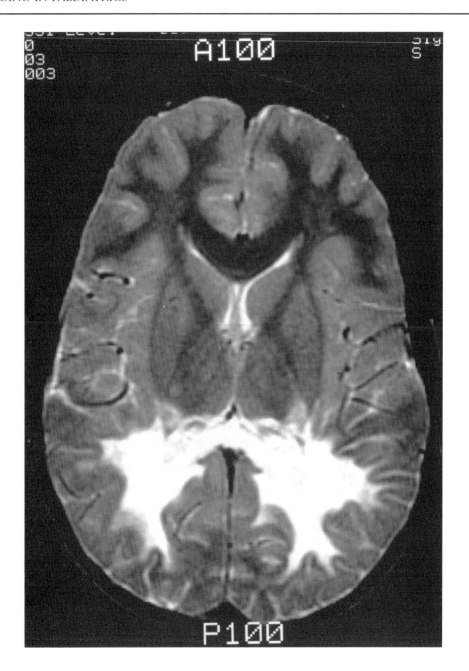

What is the diagnosis, confirmed on this axial T2 MRI brain scan, in a 9-year-old boy with behavioural change and progressive gait disturbance?

Adrenoleucodystrophy

There is symmetric abnormal hyperintense T2 signal in the white matter of the parieto-occipital regions with abnormal increased signal crossing the midline in the splenium of the corpus callosum. Compare the normal hypointense (darker) T2 signal in the white matter of the frontal lobes with the abnormal signal posteriorly.

Adrenoleucodystrophy is an X-linked disorder which results in demyelination and necrosis of the CNS white matter, and adrenal failure. The neurologic manifestations usually precede symptoms of adrenal involvement and are relentlessly progressive. Although there are several sub-types, the most common form presents in boys between the ages of 5 and 10 years. Symptoms include homonymous hemianopsia evolving to blindness with behavioural changes progressing to mental retardation and dementia. Gait disturbances with clumsiness and incoordination lead ultimately to severe ataxia and spastic quadriplegia.

Abnormalities can be evident on CT brain scans but MRI better defines the abnormal white matter in the occipital regions, with the process ultimately extending to the remaining parts of the cerebral hemispheres, brain stem, cerebellum, and long white matter tracts of the spinal cord. MRI is the best imaging modality for the assessment of the many inherited metabolic brain disorders which include the leucodystrophies.

van der Knaap, M. S. and Valk, J. (1991). The MR spectrum of peroxisomal disorders. *Neuroradiology*, 33, 30–7.

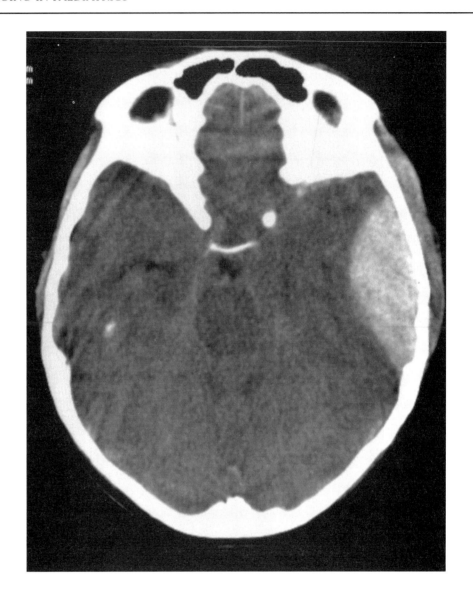

What is the diagnosis on this non-enhanced CT brain scan?

Acute extradural (epidural) haematoma

There is a high density mass lesion in the left temporoparietal region with a convex medial border, typical of acute accumulation of blood in the extradural space. There is soft tissue swelling of the scalp overlying the haematoma and a skull vault fracture was evident on specific bone window images. Increased intracranial pressure is manifest by compression of the CSF containing cisterns surrounding the brain stem.

Acute extradural (epidural) haematomas are usually caused by direct trauma resulting in tears in the middle meningeal artery in adolescents and adults and often by tears in emissary veins or venous sinuses in younger children. Unlike in adults, the classic lucid interval between the head injury and the onset of a depressed level of consciousness is often lacking, and acute extradural haematomas may occur without an associated skull fracture. An extradural haematoma is a neurosurgical emergency requiring immediate drainage.

Dhellemnes, P., Legaine, J. P., Christiaens, J. L., *et al.* (1985). Traumatic extradural haematomas in infancy and childhood. *J. Neurosurg.* **62**, 861–4.

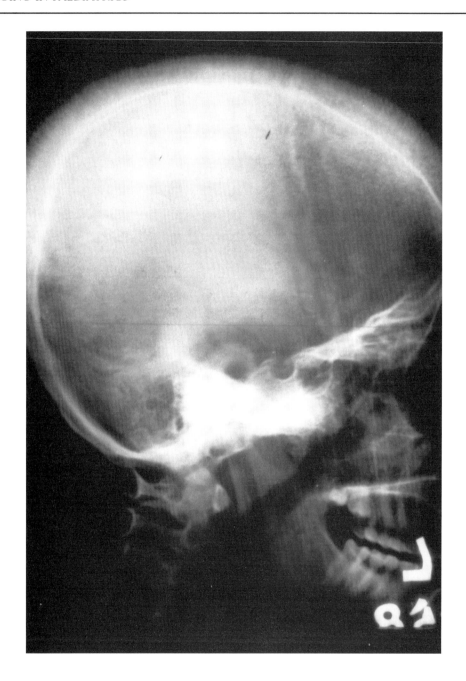

This is the lateral skull radiograph in a child of Mediterranean descent who has chronic anaemia. What is the diagnosis?

Thalassaemia

There is widening of the diploic space due to extramedullary haemopoiesis with thickening of the skull vault despite thinning of the inner and outer tables; the skull vault has a 'hair-on-end' appearance.

The thalassaemia syndromes result from reduced synthesis of one or more of the globin polypeptide chains that combine to form haemoglobin. The inevitable chronic haemolytic anaemia leads to compensatory hyperplasia of haemopoietic tissue. There is hepato-splenomegaly and marrow enlargement in the skeleton. Expansion of the marrow space may be complicated by bone pain and pathologic fractures. Bilirubin gallstones are common in adolescence.

On skull radiographs, thickening of the vault is present due to marrow hyperplasia. The classic 'hair-on-end' appearance is seen because the trabeculae run perpendicular to the bony cortex. With the exception of the ethmoidal sinuses, the paranasal air sinuses are usually poorly pneumatized. In the long bones, the cortex is thinned, the trabeculae are reduced in number and bone modelling may be impaired. Rib lesions are frequent, and include cortical thinning, osteoporosis, localized lucencies, and a pseudotumour appearance of the posterior ribs due to extramedullary haemopoiesis. Thalassaemia is one of the causes of a so-called Erlenmeyer flask deformity of the distal femora due to abnormal modelling.

Singcharoen, T. (1989). Unusual long bone changes in thalassaemia: findings on plain radiography and computed tomography. *Br. J. Radiol.*, **62**, 168–71.

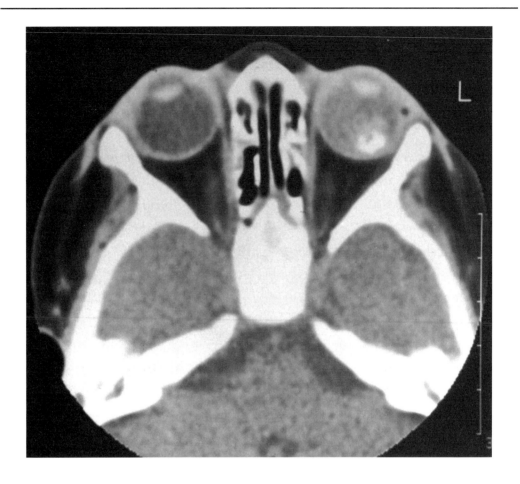

What abnormality is present in the left globe in this two year old with leucocoria?

Retinoblastoma

There is dense calcification evident in the posterior aspect of the left vitreous humour, with diffusely increased attenuation present throughout the posterior chamber on the left side. The right globe is normal.

Retinoblastoma is the most common intraocular tumour in childhood. Approximately 85% of tumours present before three years of age. Growth typically occurs into the vitreous humour with spread into the subretinal space occasionally leading to retinal detachment. Most cases are sporadic in nature with unilateral involvement but a hereditary type with autosomal dominant inheritance can result in bilateral retinoblastomas. Haemotogenous metastases to bone, lungs, and brain are known complications.

Ultrasonography of the orbit can demonstrate an intraocular mass with or without retinal detachment. CT is highly sensitive in detecting the calcification frequently found in these neoplasms; it is superior to sonography in demonstrating direct extension to the optic nerve and can also assess intracranial spread of tumour. MRI is inferior to CT in the detection of calcification and for this reason CT is probably the best imaging modality for evaluating retinoblastomas.

Azarkia, B., Naheedy, M. H., Elias, D. A. *et al.* (1987). Optic nerve tomours: role of magnetic resonace imaging and computed tomography. *Radiol. Clin. North Am.*, **25**, 561–99.

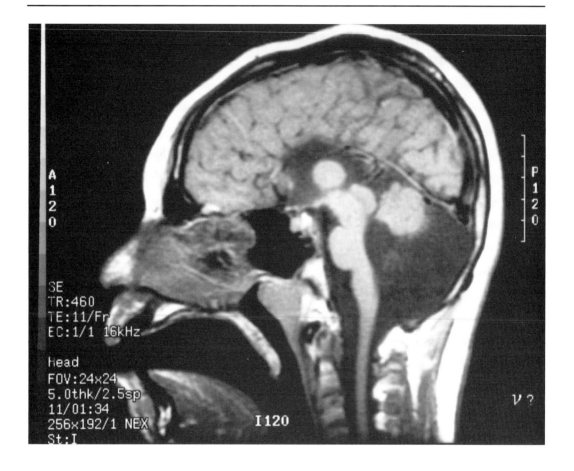

What two congenital anomalies are visible on the sagittal T1 weighted MRI brain scan?

1. Agenesis of the corpus callosum
2. Inferior cerebellar vermian agenesis (Dandy–Walker variant)

There is complete absence of the corpus callosum, which is normally seen on midline sagittal T1 images as a thick band of myelinated white matter of increased T1 signal relative to the grey matter. The inferior cerebellar vermis is replaced by an excess of CSF in the posterior fossa communicating directly with an enlarged fourth ventricle.

The Dandy–Walker syndrome comprises cystic dilatation of the fourth ventricle, enlargement of the posterior fossa, cerebellar vermian agenesis and supratentorial hydrocephalus. In a Dandy–Walker variant there is partial vermian agenesis, a normal posterior fossa and hydrocephalus is absent.

Other congenital malformations frequently found in association with agenesis of the corpus callosum include ectopic grey matter and lipoma of the corpus callosum. The majority of patients have mental retardation and a seizure disorder is present in approximately 50%.

In normal individuals the medial cerebral sulci and gyri parallel the corpus callosum and cingulate gyrus. Callosal agenesis can be suspected on cerebral ultrasound by observing that the medial sulci and gyri have a radial pattern converging on the roof of an elevated third ventricle through the area normally occupied by the corpus callosum. On coronal ultrasound and axial CT scanning, other typical findings include wide separation of the lateral ventricles which appear abnormally parallel in configuration, an elevated third ventricle, enlarged trigones, and occipital horns of the lateral ventricles (colpocephaly). MRI, by imaging in the sagittal plane, is ideal for demonstrating absence of the corpus callosum, and is superior to the other imaging modalities in depicting the other associated congenital anomalies.

Barkovich, A. J. and Norman, D. (1988). Anomalies of the corpus callosum: correlation with further anomalies of the brain. *A.J.N.R.*, **9**, 493–501.

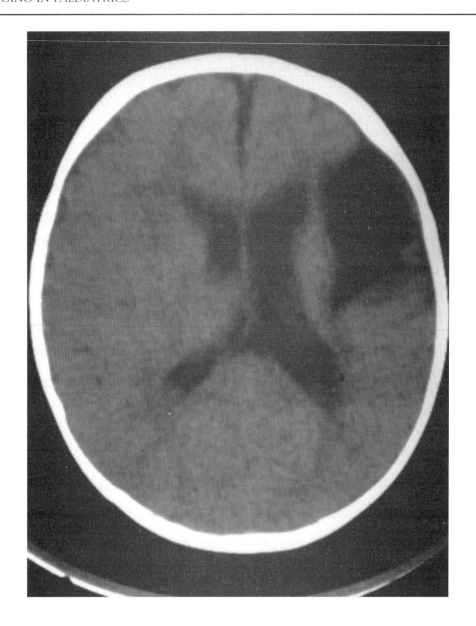

What abnormality is evident on this CT brain scan in a 7 year old with long-standing hemiplegia?

Cerebral infarction

There is a well-defined almost square-shaped area of low attenuation in the left fronto-temporal region with associated dilatation of the left lateral ventricle indicating focal cerebral atrophy. These appearances are typical of a mature infarct in the distribution of the left middle cerebral artery with liquefaction necrosis. The aetiology of this cerebrovascular accident was not conclusively proven, and may have occurred in the perinatal period.

Neonatal or perinatal stroke, typically in a full-term infant, commonly results in middle cerebral artery territory ischaemia. It can be due to stretching of the cervical carotid artery due to hyperextension or forceps injury, or may be secondary to vascular occlusion from placental emboli. Seizures rather than a focal neurologic deficit are the usual presenting symptom. Unlike older patients, hemiplegia may only become apparent long after the initial insult.

Paediatric stroke has an annual incidence of approximately 2.5 per 100 000 children. A wide variety of disorders can result in paediatric cerebrovascular accidents such as trauma, meningitis, vascular dysplasia, coagulopathy, cardiac, and metabolic diseases. Up to 75% of ischaemic events in children are found to be associated with specific conditions known to have an increased stroke risk. The frequency of ischaemic and haemorrhagic strokes is approximately equal with haemorrhagic lesions more likely to result from trauma, aneurysm, or a vascular malformation.

CT performed very soon after infarction may be normal and can remain normal for up to 48 hours, although reduced attenuation of the area of ischaemia is often evident within four to six hours. Over time, volume loss and encephalomalacia mark the site of ischaemic insult on both CT and MRI.

Lanska, M. J., Lanska, D. J., Horwitz, S. J. et al. (1991). Presentation clinical course and outcome of childhood stroke. Pediatr. Neurol., 7, 334–41.

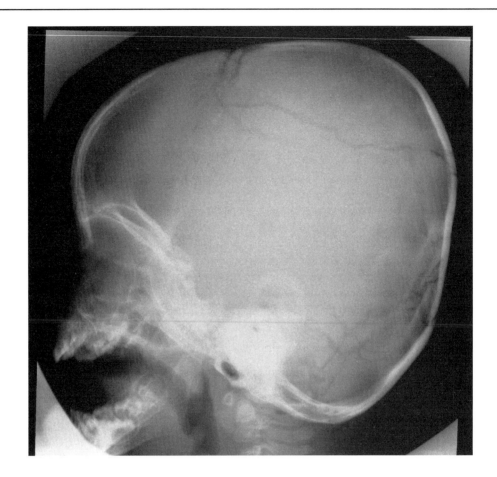

What abnormalities are visible on the lateral skull radiograph?

Bilateral parietal bone fractures

Two linear lucencies, typical of fractures, are seen traversing the parietal bones. The linear fractures extend anteriorly to each coronal suture indicating bilateral parietal bone fractures. The bilaterality of these fractures was confirmed on an AP radiograph.

Normal sutures are generally recognizable as radiolucencies in the correct anatomical position for cranial vault sutures and by their characteristic serrated edges. Fractures on the other hand usually appear as linear shadows away from the site of normal sutures, and in the acute phase are often associated with overlying soft tissue swelling. Although the presence of soft tissue swelling suggests a recent injury, as skull fractures can persist unchanged radiographically for months, accurate dating of these fractures is generally not possible. Skull fractures may be of the simple linear type, diastatic (with abnormal suture separation), comminuted, or depresssed. Significant trauma to a child's skull vault is necessary to produce a fracture such as in a road traffic accident or falling from a height (probably greater than 1 metre) on to a hard surface. A fall from a bed or sofa rarely results in a skull fracture.

Fractures of the cranial vault can result from accidental or non-accidental injury. Certain patterns of injury are more suggestive of child abuse e.g. fractures crossing the sagittal suture, occipital or multiple fractures, or fractures greater than 5 mm in width. An unexplained fracture of the calvarium in an infant is an indication for a skeletal survey to exclude other unexpected or healing fractures which would increase the likelihood of non-accidental injury.

Leventhal, J. M., Thomas, S. A., Rosenfield, N. S., and Markowitz, R. I. (1993). Fractures in young children. Distinguishing child abuse from unintentional injuries. *Am. J. Dis. Child.*, **147**, 87–92.

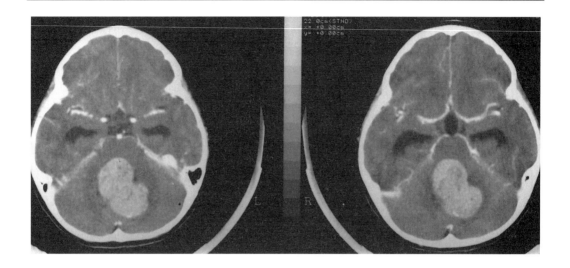

This child presented with vomiting and papilloedema. What are the two most likely diagnoses from the enhanced CT examination?

1. Medulloblastoma
2. Ependymoma

There is homogenous enhancement of a large midline mass lesion in the posterior fossa. Note normal enhancement of the basilar and middle cerebral arteries. A dilated third ventricle and temporal horns of the lateral ventricles are evident on these sections.

Medulloblastoma and ependymoma are the two common midline mass lesions that occur in the posterior fossa in children. Cerebellar astrocytoma is the other common childhood posterior fossa tumour but this tumour is usually located eccentrically in a cerebellar hemisphere. Medulloblastomas and ependymomas may be indistinguishable on CT or MRI. MR imaging is superior to CT in the evaluation of the posterior fossa as dense bone artefact from the skull base on CT can obscure detail. Many of these children, however, present as an emergency with raised intracranial pressure such that CT is commonly the first imaging study performed.

Medulloblastomas are relatively common neoplasms accounting for up to 25% of paediatric intracranial tumours. They arise in the cerebellar vermis and are typically large midline mass lesions at presentation which show homogenous enhancement after contrast administration. Leptomeningeal seeding to elsewhere in the brain and spinal cord is best assessed with gadolinium-enhanced MRI. Ependymomas may be benign or malignant and arise in the wall of the fourth ventricle. Cystic and calcific foci within the tumour are more common with ependymomas than medulloblastomas but the enhancement pattern of both neoplasms can be similar. Supratentorial hydrocephalus is frequently found in association with both tumours.

Mueller, D. P., Moore, S. A., Sato, Y., and Yuh, W. T. (1992). MRI spectrum of medulloblastoma. *Clin. Imaging*, **16**, 250–5.

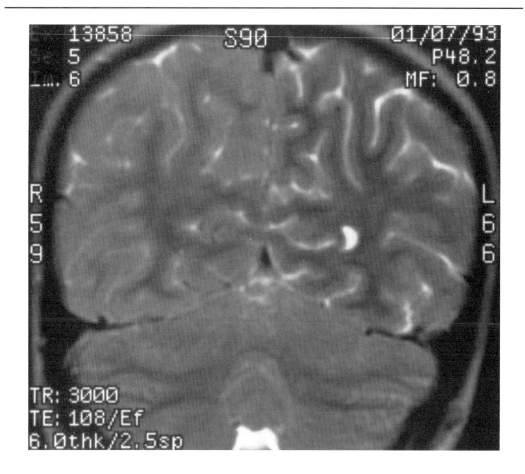

This is a coronal T2 weighted MR image of the brain. What is the diagnosis in this child with fever and a depressed level of consciousness?

Encephalitis: secondary to herpes simplex

There is poor definition of the sulci and gyri in the right supratentorial brain with abnormal signal predominantly affecting the grey matter of the parieto-occipital region on this image. The left cerebral hemisphere and the cerebellum are normal.

The congenital form a herpes encephalitis is part of the TORCH (toxoplasmosis, rubella, cytomegalovirus, and herpes simplex) syndrome and generally results in microcephaly, mental retardation, and profound neurological impairment. Herpes simplex encephalitis is usually due to the Type II virus in neonates and infants whereas Type I infections predominate in older children. After the neonatal period patients commonly present with fever and acute alteration in consciousness. Seizure and motor deficits are frequent.

The characteristic abnormality on CT scanning is low attenuation in the medial temporal lobe but CT can often be normal at presentation. MRI is more sensitive in the detection of encephalitic changes than CT, typically showing abnormal T2 signal in the temporal lobes but any part of the supratentorial brain can be affected. Herpetic encephalitis has a tendency to affect predominantly the grey matter but can progress to widespread oedema with or without haemorrhagic changes. Gyriform calcification at grey–white matter junctions is a well-recognized sequel to herpes simplex encephalitis in neonates and infants. The mortality in untreated herpes encephalitis can be as high as 70%. Early anti-viral treatment is required but may not prevent severe brain damage and subsequent cerebral atrophy.

Olson, L. C., Buesher, El, Artenstein, M. S. *et al.* (1993) Herpes virus infections of the central nervous system. *N.E.J.M.*, **277**, 1271–7.

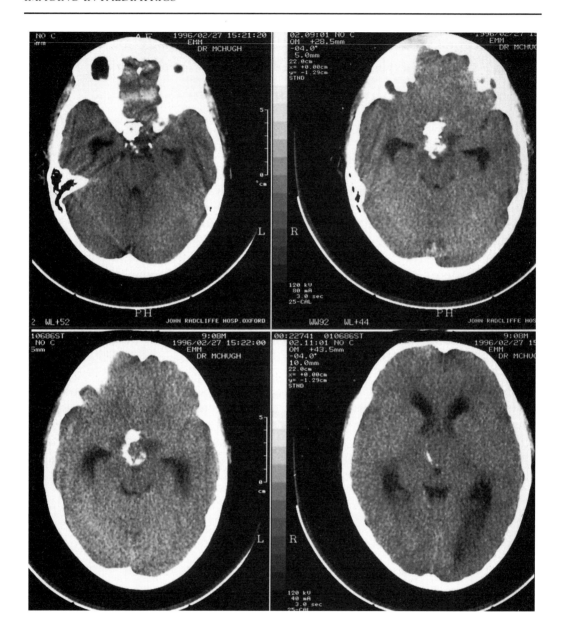

Unenhanced CT sections through the suprasellar region in a 12-year-old boy with growth retardation and headaches. What is the diagnosis?

Craniopharyngioma

There is a large calcified suprasellar mass lesion evident with calcification seen in the inferior aspect of the tumour extending into the pituitary fossa region. Superiorly the mass is obstructing the third ventricle resulting in hydrocephalus with dilatation of the lateral ventricles (including the temporal horns).

Craniopharyngiomas, which are the most common suprasellar tumours in childhood, are histologically benign, slow-growing lesions. Craniopharyngiomas arise from Rathke's pouch which is an embryonic tract between the pharynx and pituitary gland. Clinical presentation is variable with signs of raised intracranial pressure, visual field defects, and hypothalamic-pituitary dysfunction (growth retardation, delayed puberty, diabetes insipidus) commonly noted.

The suprasellar mass can be quite large and locally invasive making complete resection difficult. Extension into the sella turcica or hypothalamic regions in particular is frequent. Craniopharyngiomas are usually cystic, or partially cystic and solid. Calcification is frequently present and enhancement of the wall or capsule of the mass may be seen after intravenous contrast administration. Despite a low sensitivity in the detection of calcification, MRI is superior to CT in the evaluation of craniopharyngiomas because of its ability to image in the coronal and sagittal planes thereby allowing involvement or displacement of adjacent structures such as the optic chiasm to be more easily identifiable.

Mark, R. J., Lutge, W. R., Shimizu, K. T. *et al.* (1995). Craniopharyngioma: treatment in the CT and MR imaging era. *Radiology*, **197**, 195–8.

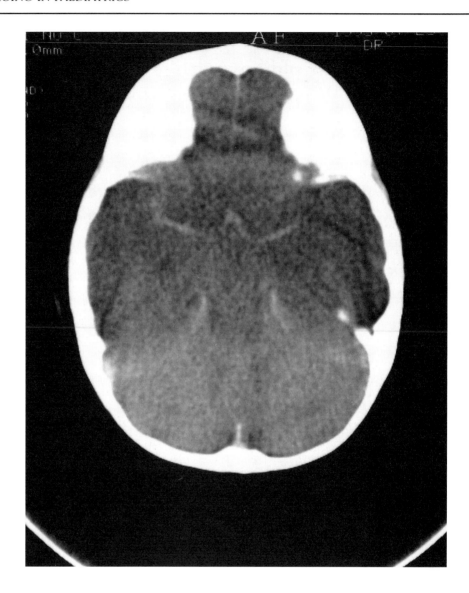

This child suffered a prolonged cardio-respiratory arrest. What abnormality is evident on CT?

Hypoxic-ischaemic encephalopathy

There is diffuse low attenuation of the supratentorial brain with loss of the normal differentiation between grey and white matter. Compare the normal cerebellum to the rest of the supratentorial brain which should be of similar attenuation. In addition, cerebral oedema with increased intra-cranial pressure is evident resulting in obliteration of the normal CSF containing basal cisterns surrounding the brain stem.

In infants with an open fontanelle, cranial sonography can occasionally show cerebral oedema manifesting as diffusely increased echogenicity in the white matter with compression of the lateral ventricles. CT, however, is more sensitive in the detection of diffuse cerebral oedema often demonstrating in severe cases unusual preminence of the cerebellum—a 'white cerebellum' or *reversal sign* of hypoxic-ischaemic encephalopathy. This appearance can be produced by a variety of hypoxic insults to the paediatric brain including the non-accidental, shaken baby syndrome. Regional redistribution of cerebral blood flow occurs as a result of the hypoxia with preferred perfusion of the brain stem and cerebellum and often of the basal ganglia also. Consequently these structures maintain a more normal attenuation contrasted against the darker background formed by the oedematous cerebrum. Surviving patients with these findings on CT often have profound neurologic deficits with severe developomental delay.

Han, B. K., Towbin, R. B., De Courten-Myers, G. *et al.* (1989). Reversal sign on CT: effect of anoxic/ischaemic cerebral injury in children. *Am. J. Neuroradiol.*, **10**, 1191–8.

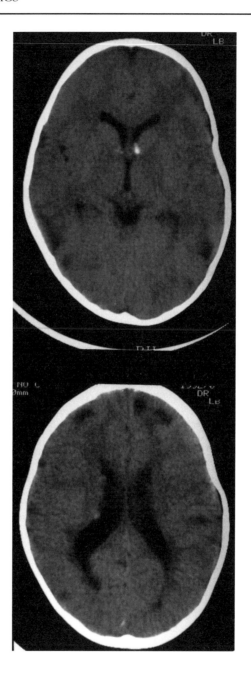

Two unenhanced CT sections through the brain in a three year old with seizures and mental retardation. What is the diagnosis?

Tuberous sclerosis

Small foci of increased attenuation due to calcified tubers at the junction between the third and lateral ventricles i.e. at the formina of Monro, are present bilaterally. The section through a higher level also shows one non-calcified subependymal nodule in the wall of the right lateral ventricle, and the low attenuation foci in the frontal lobes are due to cortical hamartomas.

Tuberous sclerosis is characterized by mental retardation, seizures, and adenoma sebaceum. The rash of adenoma sebaceum which occurs in a butterfly distribution over the face often does not appear until after six years of age. Subungal fibromas, cystic bone changes, cardiac rhabdomyomas, and hamartomas elsewhere are frequently found in association. Approximately half of cases result from autosomal dominant inheritance with the rest being due to new mutations.

Subependymal nodules are the most characteristic CT manifestation of tuberous sclerosis. The nodules or tubers tend to be small, round, and multiple and generally calcify after 18 months to two years of age. Tubers do not normally enhance after intravenous contrast administration but lesions at the foramen of Monro have the propensity to undergo malignant change into giant cell astrocytomas with rapid enlargement and variable contrast enhancement. Cortical hamartomas which are thought to be epileptogenic foci tend to be larger than the subependymal tubers, although malignant degeneration of cortical lesions is rare. Cortical tubers are often difficult to identify on CT examinations but are much more readily apparent on MRI as areas of abnormal T2 signal.

Webb, D. W. and Osborne, J. P. (1995). Tuberous sclerosis. *Arch. Dis. Child.*, **72**, 471–4.

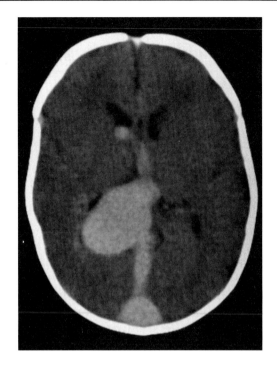

(a)

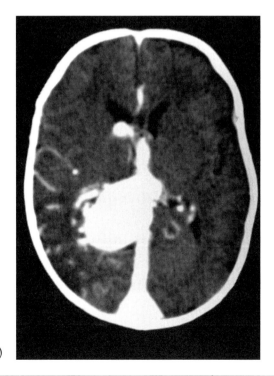

(b)

What lesion is present on the (a) unenhanced, and (b) enhanced CT brain scans in this neonate with congestive cardiac failure?

Vein of Galen malformation

There is marked globular dilatation of the vein of Galen with associated enlargement of the straight sinus. These vascular structures show intense enhancement after intravenous contrast administration. The lateral ventricles are of normal size.

The so-called vein of Galen 'aneurysm' is a commonly used misnomer for extensive enlargement of the vein of Galen resulting from a congenital arterio-venous malformation. Dilatation of the lateral ventricles is usually present due mainly to compression of the aqueduct of Sylvius by the enlarged vein of Galen. Severe arterio-venous shunting in neonates results in congestive heart failure but milder degrees of arterio-venous shunting may be well tolerated in young infants and can manifest solely with hydrocephalus.

Cerebral ultrasound can easily confirm the presence of a large mass due to vein of Galen dilatation, the vascular nature of which can be confirmed by Doppler examination. Any associated hydrocephalus will be readily apparent. CT or MRI should be performed subsequently to assess the venous sac, hypertrophied arteries, and enlarged draining veins further. The cerebral parenchyma should be carefully evaluated as anoxic cerebral injury is a frequent association. Provided there is no irreparable cerebral damage, embolisation of the feeding arteries via an arterial route is the treatment of choice.

Lasjaunias, P., Garcia-Monaco, R. and Rodesch, G. (1991). Vein of Galen malformation: endovascular management of 43 cases. *Child's Nervous System*, **7**, 360–7.

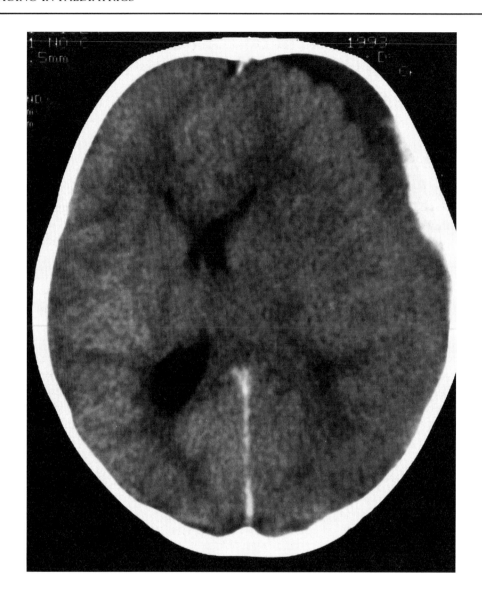

This is an unenhanced CT brain scan of a five month old. What is the abnormality?

Acute on chronic subdural haematoma

The right cerebral hemisphere is essentially normal with preservation of the grey–white interface and CSF of normal low attenuation in the right lateral ventricle. There is a left-sided extra-cerebral collection comprising intermediate attenuating fluid (relative to CSF) due to old blood, and bright or high attenuating fluid secondary to fresh haemorrhage. (The acute blood is difficult to distinguish from the skull vault but note the apparent thickness of the left vault compared to the right). The crescent-shaped layering of this collection over much of the hemisphere is typical of a subdural haematoma. In addition there is oedema in the hemisphere with compression of the left lateral ventricle and midline shift.

The terms 'density' and 'attenuation' are used interchangeably in CT reporting—darker areas are best referred to as areas of low attenuation and brighter areas as high attenuation. Subdural haematomas are caused by tearing of veins that traverse the subdural space. Severe trauma is necessary to produce a subdural haematoma in normal infants. In the absence of documented trauma, the possibility of non-accidental injury (the shaken baby syndrome) should be entertained particularly if there are other unexplained injuries as subdural haematomas are a relatively frequent manifestation of child abuse.

Cohen, R. A., Kaufman, R. A., Myers, P. A. *et al.* (1986). Cranial computed tomography in the abused child with head injury. *Am. J. Roentgenol.*, **146**, 97–102.

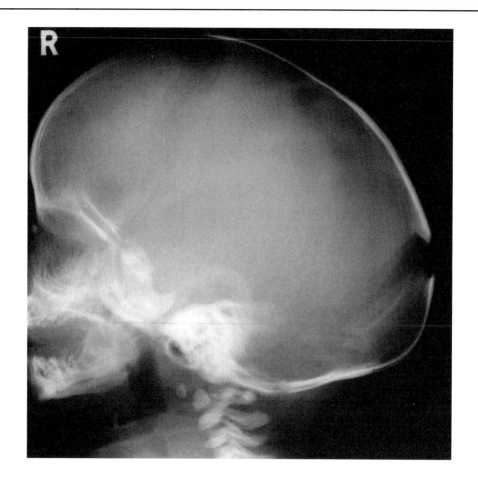

What is causing the abnormality of skull shape in this infant?

Sagittal suture synostosis

The skull vault has an elongated anteroposterior diameter resulting in a boat-shaped appearance or scaphocephaly. Note the widened coronal and lambdoid sutures.

Craniosynostosis results from premature fusion of one or multiple cranial vault sutures. Growth continues at the other patent sutures leading to an abnormal skull shape. Premature sutural fusion may occur as an isolated defect or part of a broader pattern of malformations. Premature sutural closure may involve all or part of the suture—absence of the normal suture will be evident on plain radiographs often with a dense sclerotic line replacing all or part of the involved suture.

Scaphocephaly due to sagittal suture synostosis in the most common form (55%). The skull is narrow and elongated. Bilateral coronal suture synostosis results in a short anterior cranial fossa, a narrow sagittal diameter to the skull, proptosis, and bilateral Harlequin orbit deformities on AP radiographs. Coronal suture synostosis occurs in both Apert's and Crouzon's syndromes which are inherited as autosomal dominant conditions. Premature closure of the metopic suture between the frontal bones results in a triangular, pointed forehead, or trigonocephaly. Plagiocephaly is a commonly used descriptive term for an asymmetric skull shape. Such asymmetry may merely be positional in origin and of no clinical consequence but when due to synostosis is generally secondary to unilateral fusion of a coronal or lambdoid suture.

Benson, M. L., Oliverio, P. J., Yue, N. C., and Zinreich, S. J. (1996). Primary craniosynostosis: imaging features. *Am. J. Roentgenol.*, **166**, 697–703.

Bibliography

1. Silverman, F. N. and Kuhn, J. P. (1993). *Caffey's pediatric X-ray diagnosis. An integrated imaging approach.* 9th edition. Volumes 1 and 2. Mosby, St. Louis.
2. Carty, H., Brunelle, F., Shaw, D., and Kendall, B. (1994). *Imaging children.* Volumes 1 and 2. Churchill-Livingstone, Edinburgh.
3. Keats, T. E. and Smith, T. H. (1977). *An atlas of normal developmental roentgen anatomy.* Year Book Medical Publishers, Chicago.
4. Siegel, M. J. (1992). *Pediatric sonography.* Raven Press, New York.
5. Cohen, M. D. and Edwards, M. K. (1990). Magnetic resonance imaging of children. BC Decker, Philadelphia.
6. Stringer, D. A. (1989). Pediatric gastrointestinal imaging. BC Decker, Toronto.
7. Taybi, H. and Lachman, R. S. (1990). *Radiology of syndromes, metabolic disorders and skeletal dysplasias.* 3rd edition. Year Book Medical Publishers, Chicago.
8. Treves, S. T. (1995). *Pediatric nuclear medicine.* 2nd edition. Springer-Verlag, Berlin.
9. Barkovich, A. J. (1994). *Pediatric neuroimaging.* 2nd edition. Raven Press, New York.
10. Swischuk, L. E. (1994). *Emergency imaging of the acutely ill or injured child.* Williams and Wilkins, Baltimore.

Appendix I: Approach to the paediatric chest radiograph

1. Technical factors

Check patient name, left or right side markers, date of X-ray.

Note whether the radiograph was taken in the supine or erect position.

Exposure: With adequate exposure of the radiograph the vertebrae can be seen clearly through the heart.

Rotation: Symmetry of the anterior rib lengths is generally more reliable than the position of the clavicles.

Inspiration: A film taken on expiration shows eight or less posterior ribs above the diaphragm. Ideally, nine or ten ribs should be seen. Compare with previous films if available.

2. Catheters, tubes, lines, and drains

Evaluate the siting and possible associated complications of any catheters or tubes.

3. Heart—size and shape

Assess heart size. If cardiomegaly present—which chamber dilated?

(LV enlargement displaces the cardiac apex inferiorly. RV enlargement elevates the apex. LA dilatation may splay the carina. Echocardiography necessary to diagnose most congenital lesions and pericardial effusion.)

4. Mediastinum—widened or narrow

Assess major airways and position of the aortic arch.

Hilar adenopathy?

5. Lungs

Assess lung volume—reduced or hyperinflated?

Focal lung pathology e.g. lobar consolidation—which lobe affected.

Other infiltrates, atelectasis, pulmonary oedema, pleural effusion?

Assess pulmonary vascularity—normal and symmetrical; increased or decreased.

6. Miscellaneous

Check 'hidden' areas—lung apex, behind the heart, upper abdomen.
Assess the skeleton—ribs, clavicles, humeri, and vertebrae.

N.B. Compare with previous films. Interesting films that are missing are usually in a paediatrician's office or car—they are never misfiled by radiology!

Index